Clinical Concepts for COTAs

Vicki Smith, MBA, OTR/L

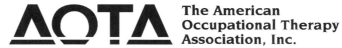

AOTA The American
Occupational Therapy
Association, Inc.

Clinical Concepts for COTAs is produced by the American Occupational Therapy Association. Issues of *Clinical Concepts for COTAs* may not be reproduced in whole or in part by any means without permission. For information, address The American Occupational Therapy Association, Inc., 4720 Montgomery Lane, PO Box 31220, Bethesda, MD 20824-1220.

The American Occupational Therapy Association, Inc. Mission Statement

The mission of the American Occupational Therapy Association is to support a professional community for members, and to develop and preserve the viability and relevance of the profession. The organization serves the interest of its members, represents the profession to the public, and promotes access to occupational therapy services.

Disclaimers

"This publication is designed to provide accurate and authoritative information in regard to the subject matter covered. It is sold or distributed with the understanding that the publisher is not engaged in rendering legal, accounting, or other professional services. If legal advice or other expert assistance is required, the services of a competent professional should be sought."

—*From the Declaration of Principles jointly adopted by the American Bar Association and a Committee of Publishers and Associations*

It is the objective of the American Occupational Therapy Association to be a forum for free expression and interchange of ideas. The opinions expressed by the contributors to this work are their own and not necessarily those of either the editors or the American Occupational Therapy Association.

AOTA Director of Nonperiodical Publications: Frances E. McCarrey
AOTA Managing Editor of Nonperiodical Publications: Mary C. Fisk
Text design by World Composition Services, Inc.
Cover design by Paul A. Platosh

ISBN 1-56900-093-X

Printed in the United States of America

Dedication

This book is dedicated to my husband David and our two beautiful daughters, Amber and Amy. Thank you for your love and patience.

My sincere thanks to all the students, clinicians, and colleagues who have taught me and inspired the ideas and concepts for this workbook. My special thanks to Vidya B. Kudva, MD, and Sue Hill.

Vicki Smith, MBA, OTR/L

Contents

Contributing Author

Harriet Ann Backhaus received her Certificate for Occupational Therapy Assistant from William-Woods/Westminster College in Fulton, Missouri, in 1976, and her Bachelor of Arts in Elementary Education in 1971. Harriet received her master's degree in gerontology from Webster University in St. Louis, Missouri, in 1992. Her entire career has been spent in clinical work in geriatric rehabilitation. She has been laboratory instructor for Washington University Program in Occupational Therapy in St. Louis. She was coursemaster for the OTA program at Meramec Community College in St. Louis from 1984 to 1989. She remains on the advisory board for Meramec Community College. Currently she is an adjunct faculty member in the OT program at Maryville University in St. Louis, and staff COTA for Associated Rehab/Rehab Choice in St. Louis, based at Sherbrooke Village Skilled Nursing facility in St. Louis County. Harriet received the Roster of Honor from AOTA in 1994. She served as a member of the former AOTCB committee for 6 years. She is a member of the Speaker's Bureau for the Alzheimer's Association in St. Louis.

Preface

Students and educators of occupational therapy face many challenges in completing the clinical practicum education requirements for the transition between student and professional. Students frequently are overwhelmed by the vast amount of information that is introduced the first few weeks of a clinical practicum and the difficulty of relating classroom skills to actual practice. Fieldwork supervisors often feel that students know very little about the field they have studied in the classroom because of the difficulties students have in adjusting to actual clinical practice. Accordingly, fieldwork educators' goals are to prepare students for the field and to bridge this gap.

This workbook is designed to aid in the transition from occupational therapy classroom education to occupational therapy clinical practice. The workbook has three goals:

❏ to make the OTA student aware of the components of the occupational therapy process as directed by the OTR, as well as the responsibilities involved in being a COTA. It is important to realize that the OTR does have ultimate responsibility both legally and professionally for the COTA's treatment implementation

❏ to introduce and reinforce several concepts commonly faced in the clinical education process: evaluating, goal writing, engaging in an interdisciplinary approach to treatment planning and delivery, patient care, discharge preparation, and situational activity grading

❏ to introduce the student to the concept of the therapy services continuum available for individuals during the rehabilitation and/or habilitation process.

The introduction of these concepts in the safe environment of the classroom should help decrease students' apprehension about the upcoming fieldwork experience. The concepts are designed to begin teaching students how to develop practical clinical reasoning skills. This should provide fieldwork educators with an education continuum that will prepare students for situations similar to those faced in clinical practice.

Although this workbook was originally designed to be used in the classroom setting, many of the exercises and concepts also can be used by fieldwork supervisors to assist students in achieving specific learning objectives. This technique may reduce the anxiety that many students experience during the transition from the classroom to a professional setting.

The workbook has three chapters aimed at leading students through the practical phases of evaluation, treatment, and discharge planning relating to COTA practice. Each chapter begins with objectives that outline the emphasis of the content and each concludes with exercises. The exercises consist of case descriptions that contain common medical abbreviations and symbols, which are itemized and defined in Appendix A and Appendix B, respectively. Use of such medical terms allows students to become familiar with the type of information that they are likely to encounter in clinical practice. Throughout the workbook are several examples that require ethical considerations, which allow the students to practice forming a professional position that will later prove useful in similar situations.

The students should have their exercises evaluated but not graded. Classroom education and fieldwork education have very different student evaluation styles. Grading in the classroom relies on continuous feedback on assignments so that students can measure their progress. Fieldwork education differs in that a patient's recovery provides a measurement of progress. The fieldwork supervisor relies on this standard to evaluate students.

Accordingly, it is suggested that the students not receive a letter grade on the workbook exercises, thereby simulating the fieldwork experience. It is recommended that students receive credit for completing tasks, class participation, and discussion. Students who are permitted to evaluate their own work will build self-confidence that they can bring to clinical fieldwork.

Another important feature of this workbook is that it requires students to use resources from their prior classwork. This encourages students to integrate the knowledge they have learned in class with simulated problems that will carry over into actual clinical practice. It should be emphasized that there are no right or wrong answers. The examples are designed to help students develop logical reasoning skills and integrate a vast amount of information that will ultimately help patients establish, maintain, or regain their independence.

I hope that this workbook will provide a framework for educating and preparing the occupational therapy assistant for fieldwork training. We welcome ideas and comments from colleagues and students; these attributions will help the field of occupational therapy continue to grow and develop with pride.

Vicki Smith, MBA, OTR/L

Special Note to Students

Preparing for clinical affiliation training is a very exciting and anxious time for all students. Classroom studies give students a foundation of information that will assist them with this final education process of becoming a professional. This workbook is designed to give a preview of the types of information and situations encountered within the fieldwork affiliation and in clinical practice.

Classroom and fieldwork education are very different. In classroom education, students receive continuous feedback through grades and evaluations on assignments. In the fieldwork setting, students are given assignments relating to evaluation, treatment, continuing education, and practical treatment skills; however, the supervisor does not reinforce these tasks with a grade. The goals of this type of learning are to encourage students to develop self-confidence in their own work and to obtain reinforcement through colleague interaction, patient progress, and self-satisfaction.

Students may need stronger feedback at times to verify that they are meeting the demands of the fieldwork experience. The supervisor is the source of this feedback. Becoming assertive and asking questions are part of being a professional. Even experienced therapists continue to learn by asking questions of physicians, colleagues, and in some cases students.

Students often enter their clinical practicum with the impression that they should have learned everything in the classroom setting that will make them effective therapists. Even though the classroom can assist with setting guidelines of theory and practice, no classroom can completely prepare students to develop patient rapport, engage in treatment processing, interact with colleagues, and cope with other situations that therapists experience on a daily basis.

Because human nature and the changing health care system present too many variables to consider in a classroom situation, one of the most challenging and rewarding aspects of being therapists is learning how to be flexible and creative in dealing with human nature and medical or facility limitations.

The purpose of the clinical affiliation is to provide students with exposure to these valuable situations but in a setting in which guidance is available. The clinical affiliation is a continuation of the education started in the classroom. The student is responsible for the classroom material presented during the occupational therapy education process, and the clinical supervisor is responsible for assisting with the organization of the learned information and the practical aspects of occupational therapy practice.

From the beginning of the occupational therapy education process to registration, many individuals play a role in providing the educational requirements needed to become a therapist. Parents, counselors, teachers, school administrators, fieldwork coordinators and supervisors, facility administrators, the American Occupational Therapy Association (AOTA), and the National Board of Certification for Occupational Therapy (NBCOT) are examples. Even after the formal education is complete, students will continue to learn from colleagues, patients, clients, continuing education, students, and practice. This workbook will assist students in applying the vast amount of information they have received and in making the successful transition from student to clinician.

Editor's Note

Occupational therapy assistants use many terms to describe the individuals who receive therapeutic intervention. *Client* and *resident* are often used to avoid negative stereotypes that may be associated with the term *patient*. However, in an effort to be consistent, this workbook identifies the individuals receiving therapy as *patients* and is not meant to have a negative connotation.

CHAPTER 1

Evaluation Process

Objectives

After completing this chapter and the exercises, the student should be able to identify

❏ basic roles of the COTA/OTR relationships

❏ the types of information found in a medical chart and the relevance of the information to an occupational therapy treatment plan

❏ four elements that can assist with providing an appropriate occupational therapy evaluation

❏ various methods of gathering evaluation information to design an effective treatment plan

❏ the meaning of medical abbreviations.

Introduction

Jane is in her first week of clinical affiliation training for occupational therapy. She has been following her supervisor all week. In that time, Jane has been oriented to the department policies and evaluation forms. She has been introduced to occupational therapists, COTAs, physical therapists, speech therapists, doctors, nurses, the maintenance crew, and other personnel working in the facility. Jane's supervisor has had her observe her patients and patient evaluations. Her supervisor does everything with such ease and comfort that being a therapist looks very easy. However, Jane is worried that she will do something wrong, because she cannot remember anything she has read in the past few days.

At the end of the week, Jane is assigned a patient. Her supervisor asks her to review the medical chart and determine what information she will need to begin the patient's evaluation. Jane sits down in the busy staff office and is overwhelmed with the request. She goes to the medical chart and starts recording everything she reads. She sits back and thinks, "There is so much information here. Where do I start? What am I doing here? I don't know enough to do this."

This is a common situation faced by students on their fieldwork affiliations. The atmosphere of a clinic is very different from a school classroom. The clinic exposes the student to a great deal of distracting information that makes it difficult to stay organized and retrieve learned facts.

This chapter is designed to alleviate the anxiety of these situations. The exercises included at the end of this chapter provide the student with practical techniques to further develop skills previously learned in retrieving medical chart information and learn alternate methods of gathering evaluation information. The exercises are written with common medical abbreviations, which are defined in Appendix A, to familiarize the student with their uses.

Section I   Becoming Part of the OTR/COTA Team

During a patient's evaluation process the role of the OTR is to plan the evaluation, to administer standardized and nonstandardized tests, and to analyze the data (Hopkins & Smith, 1983). The role of the COTA is to assist the OTR in collecting the data as determined by the OTR. These tasks can include administering interest checklists or activity configurations and summarizing the information in written form, or observing patients in functional situations and reporting on activities of daily living (ADL) tasks involving various performance components, such as coordination and strength (Ryan, 1993b).

The OTR has expertise in assessing and interpreting data, and COTAs have the knowledge to carry out treatment plans and, with good observation skills, to monitor the patient's progress. OTRs and COTAs work together to make a good team.

The COTA should be present during the OTR's evaluation of the patient. This may not be possible if the OTR does the evaluations and the COTA does the treatments. As a student, you should be exposed to as many evaluations as possible. If you are supervised by a COTA, regularly scheduled meetings must take place with the OTR.

After the evaluation, the COTA and OTR must spend some time setting individual goals and treatment protocols. This collaboration should be noted somewhere in the OT documentation. In some situations, the daily log reflects the collaboration. This may vary with the settings.

As a COTA, you should know when to ask for assistance: when the patient is ready to move on in the treatment program and needs new goals, when the patient has shown a decrease in function, and when the patient is ready for discharge. COTAs should not have the responsibility to make these decisions on their own. With experience, a COTA can take on more decision making, but the ultimate legal responsibility remains with the OTR. Be aware of good documentation components and collaborate on the note writing with the OTR.

The COTA should be able to discuss patient progress with family and staff. Let the OTR know that these discussions are taking place and, when indicated, inform the OTR of what will be discussed.

These guidelines are meant especially for OTA students and newly graduated COTAs. With experience and the establishment of competencies, less direct supervision may be warranted. In most patient care areas, COTAs are supervised and, depending on the state licensure and third party reimbursers, guidelines may vary. The best means to achieve a good working relationship is to remember that the OTR does have final responsibility for the patient and, when good communication takes place, the team can be very effective.

For further explanation of the OTR/COTA team responsibility, refer to the current role delineation below.

Section II OTR/COTA Roles

A great deal of confusion exists regarding the role of the COTA in evaluations. In order to begin, a review of the entry-level role delineation for OTRs and COTAs is helpful. The purpose of the entry-level document is to give guidelines. Local, state, and reimbursement sources must be taken into account. Facilities and licensure regulations must be followed. The student should have an understanding of these issues before beginning the affiliation.

It is important for the OTA student to understand that the OTR has ultimate responsibility, both while as a student and when working as a COTA. Often an OTA student will have an experienced COTA as a supervisor, but both the COTA and the student are responsible to the OTR.

The OTA student may assist in the screening process. This process precedes evaluation and consists of the collection of data in which the need for occupational therapy services is ascertained. Screening is not an evaluation. The OTA student can assist by giving structured interviews, interest checklists, and employment histories. Other means of obtaining data are by observing the patient in functional settings, interviewing the patient, or reviewing the medical chart.

Often a referral is made directly to the occupational therapy department, and screening is not needed. This is when the patient is evaluated by the OTR. The OTA student can assist by reviewing the chart, interviewing the patient, performing general observations, and giving structured evaluations.

The Occupational Therapy Evaluation Process

The OTR provides a complete evaluation and treatment plan for each patient. The COTA should have a basic understanding of the evaluation process and rationale.

The *Uniform Terminology for Reporting Occupational Therapy Services* (Hopkins & Smith, 1983) provides a complete listing of areas a therapist should consider when performing an evaluation. Providing a complete evaluation according to these guidelines can be unrealistic in many cases because of time restraints; lack of the patient's endurance for the testing; or in some cases, insufficient funding to reimburse services. Nevertheless, occupational therapists should provide timely, responsible, and appropriate evaluations that reflect the patient's needs and that do not conflict with external factors that can interfere with patient recovery.

To determine whether an evaluation is appropriate, a therapist needs to consider many factors including

- ❏ diagnosis
- ❏ phase of recovery
- ❏ facility that is serving the patient
- ❏ other significant factors, including discharge plans, funding resources, past diagnoses, and other areas not related to the patient's current diagnosis.

Diagnosis

A patient's diagnosis can be a starting point for determining areas for an appropriate occupational therapy evaluation. The diagnosis indicates areas of disability the therapist should consider.

For example, a diagnosis of a cerebrovascular accident (CVA) indicates that there may be physical, cognitive, and perceptual deficits. Consequently, all these areas should be evaluated when treating a patient with a CVA diagnosis.

A hip fracture diagnosis is basically characterized by physical limitations. The evaluation for a patient with a hip fracture diagnosis should primarily focus on these limitations.

It is important to remember that understanding a patient diagnosis is only a starting point for an effective occupational therapy evaluation. The factors discussed next are of equal importance.

Phase of Recovery

The patient phase of recovery helps to determine appropriate occupational therapy evaluation areas. A patient in the acute phase of recovery may have limited endurance for activities. Medical precautions or being connected to medical equipment may prevent the patient from participating in a complete evaluation to determine his or her level of independence. A patient in an intensive care unit (ICU) seen 2 days after a CVA may be on a ventilator, intravenous (IV) drips, and an electrocardiogram (ECG) monitor with lines attached to the chest. As a consequence, the patient will not be able to tolerate a complete occupational therapy assessment, and the evaluation must be tailored to fit the needs at the patient's phase of recovery. On the other hand, a patient with a spinal cord injury, who is in a rehabilitation clinic and has been medically stable for 2 weeks, probably will be an appropriate candidate for a complete evaluation, because this type of patient is in a *later phase of recovery.*

Facility Considerations

The type of facility a patient is in also determines, to some degree, how a therapist should go about an evaluation. Patients in a hospital setting usually have very short lengths of stay and are generally more restricted by their illnesses. A nursing home also will be restricted in the therapy services it can provide because of the limited exposure the therapist has to the patients. Rehabilitation facilities usually have longer lengths of stay for the patients, and the patients generally are medically stable.

For example, if the evaluation and treatment approaches for a patient with a head injury in a hospital, nursing home, and rehabilitation clinic are compared, the length of time the patient is seen and the therapy goals will vary. In the hospital, the patient is seen when he or she is medically unstable and only for 1 to 2 weeks. In the nursing home the patient may receive treatment one time per day for 15 to 20 minutes. In the rehabilitation facility, the patient may get as much as 1½ hours of occupational therapy per day for 6 to 8 weeks.

Given these time restraints, it may be inappropriate to evaluate cooking skills, for instance, during the initial evaluation at a hospital or nursing home. However, a rehabilitation facility would be an appropriate location in which to address cooking activities.

Other Significant Factors

The therapist is responsible for reviewing each patient's previous medical and social history. This information also leads to areas appropriate for evaluation. Patients with a history of confusion and living in a nursing home and with a current diagnosis of a total hip replacement, will need to be evaluated differently than patients with the same diagnosis who live alone. Evaluating and teaching lower-extremity dressing skills to confused patients probably would be detrimental to their health, because they probably will not remember the total hip replacement precautions and may dislocate the hip prosthesis. Patients living independently would be more appropriate for lower-extremity dressing evaluation and training, because they are alert enough to maintain the precautions, and the training will allow them to maintain independence.

Reimbursement for services is one of the most difficult issues that therapists face when providing recommendations for continued treatment. This issue is a constant source of discomfort for many therapists and other professionals in all types of facilities. Both for-profit and nonprofit facilities operate within a budget, and there are times when an entire team of professionals can see the potential for recovery in a patient and yet the funding is not available to continue treatment. No words of wisdom can solve this situation; however, an effective therapist can provide services that may ease the burden of all persons involved. It is important to choose a theoretical basis of treatment that is the most effective for the patient, given funding limitations. (See Figure 1.1 for an outline of evaluation factors.)

It should be noted that the health care system provides many types of access to therapy services. Therapists should explore the discharge recommendation options for continued services. These issues are discussed further in Chapter 3, along with some practical solutions.

Section III   Relevance of Medical Chart Information

Documentation is an important part of being an occupational therapy assistant. The OTR is responsible for accurate evaluation, reevaluation, and discharge documentation of a patient. The COTA is often responsible for progress notes and daily documentation. The notes will be reviewed by many professionals for many reasons. For example, physicians will review the information the therapist provides to assist them with discharge planning. The therapist's notes can alert the physician to any change in the patient's status and provide documentation that can help support the physician's diagnosis. Together with the other professionals' input and personal medical knowledge, an informed decision can be made about further medical needs or placement of the patient.

Other professionals also will benefit from the reports that occupational therapy assistants provide. For example, a dietitian determines if the diet that he or she has prescribed for a patient is adequate. The dietitian may review the therapy reports and determine whether the patient is performing very low- or high-level activities.

Figure 1.1   Evaluation factors

Diagnosis
Phase of recovery
Facility that is serving the patient
Other significant factors (i.e., discharge plans, funding resources, past diagnoses) and other areas not related to the patient's current diagnosis.

The diet plan then would be adjusted to accommodate the patient's nutritional needs in relation to the daily activity level.

Insurance companies, quality assurance representatives, utilization review committees, and Medicare auditors also will review the occupational therapist's documentation to justify the cost of therapy services. A therapist who works well with patients and provides appropriate therapy for their recovery is not effective if reimbursement funds are lost for the health care provider because adequate documentation was not provided, and the charges are sent to the patient because insurance will not cover the cost of services.

It is also critical to remember that the written reports are legal documents. Occupational therapists are legally responsible for what they write and sign, and statements should be clear.

OTA documentation needs to be reviewed by the OTR. Progress notes may or may not be signed, depending on the situation; however, when goals are added to the treatment plan, the note should be signed. An example could be, once a month, the OTR and COTA collaborate on the progress note, and this note is signed by the OTR.

Types of Medical Chart Information

OTAs may view the chart and collect pertinent information on patients who have been referred to occupational therapy. When a therapist reviews the medical chart, there will be a great deal of information to consider before he or she is able to determine if occupational therapy services may be beneficial. Every profession and facility have different types of forms for writing evaluations and recommendations. However, four types of information are common to most reports: *subjective, objective, assessment,* and *plan* (Weed, 1971). Therapists should understand the differences among these types of information when developing an evaluation and treatment plan for a patient. Therapists are valuable members of any treatment team when they are able to identify and synthesize these types of information.

Subjective Information

Subjective information includes anything the patient states that is pertinent to his or her therapy. It is also anything the patient or patient's family says that cannot be substantiated, verified, or measured. This information is generally written in a narrative form and can include any of the following:

- ❏ patient's complaints of pain or discomfort
- ❏ prior functioning and living arrangements
- ❏ statements that may reflect the patient's mental status
- ❏ patient's statements related to his or her current functioning
- ❏ statements made by family members that are pertinent to the patient's treatment process.

An example of subjective documentation is

> Pt c/o pain in (R) hip. She indicates she lived alone before her fall and took care of herself. Pt states, "It is January 4, 1901," when asked the date. Family members indicate they have been worried lately about her living by herself. Pt indicates she wants to walk.

This information is considered subjective because the patient's and family's perceptions of the reality of what they are reporting may be distorted. Subjective information can be confused because of different types of interpretations.

For example, this patient's complaints of pain in the right hip may be related to a recent hip surgery, or they may be a result of unfamiliar stretching done during exercises in physical therapy.

The patient indicates she lives alone and takes care of herself. She could mean that she does not have a roommate in the nursing home and can dress, bathe, and take care of her own personal hygiene. However, the staff may be responsible for maintaining her medications and providing meals. In this case, do we really know how she is cognitively functioning?

She states it is 1901. Does this mean she is disoriented? What caused this problem? Has she always been this way? Is her disorientation a result of medications she is taking, or is she neurologically impaired? Perhaps she did not understand the question. Her family members have been worried about her lately because she lives alone. Is there a reason to worry, or are they feeling some guilt because they are unable to be with her all the time? ·

The patient's goal is to walk. Did she walk before, or has this been an unrealistic goal for the past 2 to 3 years? If her current diagnosis is a right lower-extremity amputation, is walking a realistic goal? Has she accepted the reality of the amputation? Does she know about, and is she a candidate for, a lower-extremity prosthesis?

Objective Information

Objective information includes any of the formal evaluation or reevaluation testing that has been performed. This also includes information that is received from a reliable source or from accurate testing procedures. Objective information is found throughout the medical chart and is collected in the clinical settings by all of the professionals involved in the individual's care. Objective information can include any of the following:

- ❏ general demographics (i.e., age, gender, race, birth date)
- ❏ past medical history (This information is classified as being received from a reliable source: physicians, social workers, and other professionals.)
- ❏ referring physician and orders from the physician
- ❏ diagnosis (This information is based on the physician's objective testing.)
- ❏ standardized tests (i.e., computed tomography [CT] scans, X rays, blood tests, and therapeutic evaluations)

❏ reports on what a patient is physically or mentally doing at the time of an evaluation as reported by a professional staff member qualified to evaluate the activities reported (e.g., "able to walk 50 feet with a walker" or "able to don/doff a shirt with minimal assistance").

Assessment Information

Assessment information is primarily opinion based on a professional's subjective and objective evaluation results. This information should reflect, summarize, and draw conclusions from the subjective and objective information only. If a conclusion is not supported by the subjective and objective information, it is not a valid assessment.

Assessment information can include any of the following:

❏ opinions that are based on the subjective and objective information researched by a professional (if issues are not addressed in the subjective and objective information, they should not appear in the assessment)
❏ the patient's physical and mental tolerance of treatment
❏ a summary of achieved goals or evaluation results (this includes progress or gains in function the patient has made since the last written report)
❏ potential for continued treatment
❏ recommended areas of focus for treatment.

Plan Information

The treatment plan is the objective intervention that a therapist will be providing and working toward to assist the patient in the recovery process. This plan is based on the information in the assessment portion of the discipline report. The plan information can include

❏ frequency of recommended treatment
❏ long-term goals (LTGs), which are an estimate of where the patient will be functionally at the end of the treatment process and how long it will take to complete the process
❏ short-term goals (STGs), which are specific problem areas that are addressed to form a logical sequence that works toward LTGs.

(See Figure 1.2 for a summary of the concepts discussed in the previous section.)

Practical Application

Complete exercises 1:1–1:4. They emphasize the concepts presented in this section by providing practical situations that students and practioners experience in clinical settings.

Figure 1.2   Types of medical chart information

Subjective:
Information that the patient states that the therapist feels is
pertinent to his or her treatment.

Objective:
Information from formal evaluations or reevaluation testing.

Assessment:
Primarily opinion based on professional subjective or objective
evaluation results.

Plan:
Objective intervention that a therapist provides and works
toward to assist the patient in the recovery process.

Section IV   Alternative Methods of Information Gathering

Medical chart review and determining the logical areas to assess are only part of an effective occupational therapy evaluation. The initial patient interview is also an important aspect. It provides an opportunity to gather information from the patient so that personal needs and desires can be incorporated into a treatment plan. The interview process allows the therapist to establish a clear understanding and purpose of the occupational therapy treatment. It also provides the patient with an opportunity to discuss the situation and to consider ideas for change (Willard & Spackman, 1983). These are essential components of the evaluation and treatment planning process.

Unfortunately, there are times when a verbal interview is not possible. For example, when a therapist is evaluating a patient who is in a coma state, or when the patient has characteristics of dementia or receptive or expressive aphasia, the interview technique is not an option. In these situations, nonverbal communication is necessary to develop a therapeutic relationship. Techniques used to establish effective working relationships in these cases are further explained in Chapter 2.

If the patient has impaired communication skills, the therapist will need to use alternative methods to gather information relating to the living situation, personality, interests, and past history. The treatment team and family can be effective sources for this information. Each member of the treatment team gathers specific details that are shared with other team members to formulate an effective treatment plan. The treatment team (see Figure 1.3) generally consists of a physician, physical therapist, occupational therapist, speech pathologist, social worker, recreation therapist, dietitian, nurse, and in some cases, a case manager.

| Figure 1.3   Treatment team | 11 |

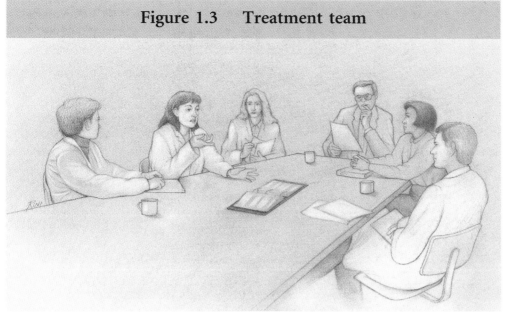

Physician

In many situations, the physician is the team leader. He or she is responsible for evaluating the patient's health and coordinating the rehabilitation process. This process includes a review of the patient's total body system. Orthopedic, neurological, internal, and external functioning of the individual are considered. The physician prescribes and regulates medications and sets precautions and limitations that the patient must follow to ensure a safe medical recovery. The physician makes referrals for therapeutic intervention and reviews therapy reports to monitor the patient's physical and cognitive recovery process (DeLisa, Martin, & Currie, 1988).

Physical Therapist

The physical therapist provides evaluations for joint range of motion, strength, endurance, and coordination. Assessments also include gross-motor skills, sitting balance, standing balance, transfers, and bed mobility. The physical therapist provides training for ambulation, including gait and wheelchair mobility. He or she also uses a variety of modalities, such as superficial and deep heat and cold, hydrotherapy, electrical stimulation, traction, and massage. Many physical therapists provide input for home evaluations and wheelchair equipment recommendations (DeLisa et al.).

Speech–Language Pathologist

The patient's communication and swallowing abilities are evaluated and treated by a speech–language pathologist. The therapist provides retraining of intraoral deficits that interfere with speech. A management program for the patients with dysphagia is devised. The therapist also provides cognitive reeducation, and evaluation and training for the use of alternative communication devices (DeLisa et al., 1988).

Social Worker

The primary role of the social worker is to facilitate communication with the patient, family, and rehabilitation team. The social worker's evaluation focuses on the patient's total living situation, including lifestyle, family, and finances. The goals are to maintain a continuing relationship with the patient and family and to provide assistance throughout the arrangement of an appropriate living situation. The social worker also addresses financial concerns that are related to the impact of the disease or disability on the patient and the entire family (DeLisa et al., 1988).

Therapeutic Recreation Specialist

The therapeutic recreation specialist provides treatment intervention that educates patients about leisure activities. He or she provides an assessment that includes the patient's needs, interests, and abilities. This information is incorporated into a program that increases the patient's leisure community access and social skills and the total spectrum of leisure capacity. The program can include adapted sports, awareness of leisure time and suitable activity choices, education about adaptive equipment that enables the individual to access leisure activities, and assistance for the patient to explore resources for postdischarge activities, such as support groups or community leisure programming (DeLisa et al., 1988; National Therapeutic Recreation Society, 1992).

Registered Dietitian

The registered dietitian is responsible for managing the patient's nutritional needs. Dietitians assess a patient's nutritional status, develop a care plan that provides the patient with adequate nutritional supplements to facilitate recovery, and monitor the use of all nutritional substances, including intravenous supplements, G-tube feedings, and food substances. The dietitian also provides nutritional counseling and education. As patients' physical activity increases or decreases, their nutritional needs will change. The dietitian monitors these changes and assists with setting restrictions that are medically necessary, such as diabetic diets (Puckett & Miller, 1988).

Nurse

The nurse and the nursing staff are the only members of the team who have the potential to monitor the patients' activity patterns 24 hours a day. As with the other disciplines, the nurse's role varies from facility to facility. The general responsibilities include providing hygiene care, managing medication distribution, watching for medication difficulties, and monitoring environmental factors. These factors include heat, noise, personal property control, sanitation, safety, and infection control. The nurse is responsible for providing interventions that minimize the effects of inactivity, such as repositioning, passive range of motion, and manipulating the environment to avoid sensory deprivation.

The nurse also provides opportunities to integrate various therapy skills into the patient's daily activities. These skills can include use of adaptive equipment for communication, mobility, or self-care. The nurse may also provide opportunities to practice learned skills. The nurse creates an evaluation and treatment plan similar to the other professional disciplines.

Case Manager

Case management is a relatively new discipline that has developed because of the national focus providing cost-effective health care services. The National Case Management Task Force Steering Committee (1991) defines case management as "an ongoing process to assure that identified clients of health and human services systems receive appropriate treatment, care, resources, and opportunities to achieve the best and most cost-effective outcome."

There are two types of case managers. One is an *internal* case manager, who is employed by the facility that is providing services to the patient. The other is an *external* case manager, who is employed by the payer or funding source for the patient. In some situations, a patient may have both types of case managers.

The role of the case manager is to provide patient advocacy and an objective assessment of an individual's needs and vulnerability by a knowledgeable professional. He or she also provides a goal-oriented plan for the rehabilitation or medical care process and documents the case as it progresses. Case managers maintain communication among the payer, patient, and family regarding any therapeutic recommendations. They coordinate and implement any accepted plan of care to maximize effective use of resources and funds (National Case Management and Task Force Steering Committee, 1991).

Section V   The COTA as a Member of the Interdisciplinary Team

The COTA will be actively involved with the other members of the treatment team. If the OTA student is not familiar with other disciplines, it is recommended that he or she spend some time observing other departments.

As an example, a patient with a head injury will be seen by all members of the team. This is referred to as an *interdisciplinary approach to treatment*. The COTA will work with nursing on following any ADL techniques taught to the patient by the COTA, with the physical therapist on mobility techniques, with the speech pathologist on communication skills, and with other members of the team during team conferences. The COTA also will work with the family members. When the patient is ready for discharge, home health can be involved to carry through with a home program. Community reentry programs also can be options.

With any patient in any setting, good communication skills among all members of the team are crucial if the patient is to be treated efficiently.

CASE STUDY: Mrs. C

Mrs. C has had a total hip replacement. Prior to her injury, she lived with her daughter. The daughter does not work and was available to help, although Mrs. C was independent in all of her ADLs. Mrs. C receives physical therapy for gait and transfer training. Mrs. C has achieved all of her physical therapy goals of independent ambulation and transfers, but because of some memory problems, she has difficulty remembering her hip precautions. The COTA has asked nursing to carry over the adapted equipment techniques taught during the occupational therapy sessions. Nursing reports that she cannot independently remember how to use the equipment.

The COTA, in collaboration with the OTR, has performed family teaching with the daughter. The COTA has shown the daughter how to help Mrs. C use the toilet and tub equipment, as well as how to use the long-handled dressing equipment. The daughter has demonstrated competency in following the precautions for total hip replacement.

The COTA informs the social worker that Mrs. C can return home with the daughter as long as the daughter gives Mrs. C assistance with bathing and dressing. Home health may not be indicated, because Mrs. C has no ambulation difficulties and she is not returning home alone.

Had Mrs. C not had anyone to care for her at home, further discussions with the team would have been necessary for possible long-term-care placement or other alternatives to ensure Mrs. C's safety.

Practical Application

Complete exercises 1:5–1:9. These emphasize the concepts presented in this section relating to interview or information gathering and evaluation process that students and practioners experience in clinical settings.

The following exercises list statements commonly found in patient records. Using the terms below, identify each statement as *subjective, objective, assessment,* or *plan information.* Briefly state the relevance of each to an occupational therapy evaluation. You are encouraged to use any occupational therapy references available.

Hint: To determine the information's relevance, imagine in each case that there are two different patients about whom nothing is known. When a piece of information is presented about one of the patients, how would that information change your approach to the patient or family members in terms of evaluation or treatment?

S = Subjective   A = Assessment
O = Objective   P = Plan

___P___   1. Example: Pt to wear forearm cast and come in for follow-up appointment and X ray in 5 weeks.

                 Relevance: The patient may need adaptive training for one-handed dressing, bathing, and ADL. Monitor and provide training for edema control and exercises for exposed joints to minimize complications that can occur secondary to decreased general use of upper extremity.

_____   2. Pt is primarily limited by ↓'d endurance for activities.
                 Relevance:

_____   3. Speech report states, "Pt shows min limitations c̄ expressive language skills."
                 Relevance:

_____   4. Ox saturation levels are 80% at rest c̄ room air.
                 Relevance:

_____   5. Pt's father reports that his daughter is a straight "A" student, very popular and outgoing, and never drinks alcohol. Reliability of the father has not been established. The pt is in hospital after a car accident while intoxicated. Records show hx of alcohol-related incidents.
                 Relevance:

—————— 6. X ray shows comminuted fx of the R tibia.
Relevance:

—————— 7. Pt nonweight-bearing 6–8 weeks on R LE and follow-up X ray in 4 weeks.
Relevance:

—————— 8. Physician report states, "Pt shows good potential for intensive rehabilitation."
Relevance:

—————— 9. CT scan of brain indicates infarct of R parietal lobe.
Relevance:

—————— 10. Student to be trained c̄ adaptive computer for completing homework assignments.
Relevance:

—————— 11. A pt who has been in the hospital for 3 days states, "I had a nice visit c̄ my sister in New York yesterday; I just got back this morning."
Relevance:

—————— 12. Nursing reports the pt does not have any problems c̄ hand-to-mouth self-feeding.
Relevance:

—————— 13. Pt to be started on Macrodantin for 10 days and follow-up c̄ urine culture.
Relevance:

—————— 14. OT report from previous facility states, Pt's primary limitation is cog. functioning, which interferes c̄ ADLs.
Relevance:

_____S_____ 1. Example: Social Services report states, Pt appears indep. c̄ all aspects of self-care.
Relevance: Provides information that can guide the evaluation process. A brief evaluation process for ADL is indicated.

_____ 2. Speech reports that the pt is not reliable for communication 2° to receptive aphasia disorder.
Relevance:

_____ 3. Pt states, "My birthday is June 15, 1899."
Relevance:

_____ 4. Recommend providing ADL training 5× per week to ↑ pt level of indep.
Relevance:

_____ 5. Nsg reports the pt appears depressed.
Relevance:

_____ 6. OT report from previous facility states, Pt requires min A for bathing and dressing 2° to ↓'d endurance.
Relevance:

_____ 7. Social Services reports that the pt shows questionable reliability for significant life hx.
Relevance:

_____ 8. Pt to be d/c'd to her home c̄ her husband as the primary caregiver.
Relevance:

_____ 9. Initiate bowel and bladder training program.
Relevance:

_____ 10. PT report states, "Pt shows poor potential for ambulation at this time."
Relevance:

_____ 11. PT reports, "Pt is able to ambulate 35 ft c̄ wheeled walker and SBA."
Relevance:

_____ 12. Pt states, "I hurt all over."
Relevance:

_____ 13. Physician report states, "Pt shows good comprehension of current limitations."
Relevance:

_____ 14. Pt states, "I want to be able to go home c̄ my wife and use my arm again."
Relevance:

_____ 15. Strength at (R) UE shows F+ at shoulder girdle, G strength at elbow flex/ext, G at wrist flex/ext, and shows 50# grip strength by OT report.
Relevance:

Complete the following exercises. Remember the treatment plans are guides for activities. Make note of other deficits identified in the occupational therapy evaluation summary and try to incorporate activities that will address them. Make sure activities are functional and purposeful.

The pt has a Dx of CVA s/p 3 days. The CT scan showed an occlusion of the internal carotid artery. Pt is currently in the ICU. Prior to this injury, pt was retired and lived with his wife independently. Other medical complications include MI s/p 6 months and IDDM. He will be seen in the ICU, followed to the acute care floor, and transferred to a rehab unit.

A. Diagnosis: CVA, occlusion of the internal carotid artery.

- ❏ Occlusion can be caused by thrombosis or embolism.
- ❏ Can produce contralateral signs: Homonymous hemianopsia, central type of facial paralysis, hemiparesis of hemiplegia, hemisensory loss, dysphagia, aphasia.
- ❏ Acute phase usually causes impairment of consciousness (drowsiness to coma).

B. Phase of recovery:

- ❏ acute; patient is medically unstable

C. Facility considerations:

- ❏ ICU environment limits therapy sessions to short periods due to medical needs and patient's medical status

D. Other significant areas:

- ❏ past medical history: MI and IDDM
- ❏ future placement plans: Transfer to acute care and then to rehab unit
- ❏ patient's functional level prior to incident

Occupational Therapy Evaluation Summary

Cognitive Status: Pt oriented × 1; he is verbally intact, shows poor sequencing for simple tasks, and is able to follow 1-step commands.

Physical Status: Pt tolerates 5–10 min of low-level activity; sitting balance @ edge of bed requires mod (A) × 1; sit ↔ supine max (A).

(R) UE Status: Pt shows min ✓ tone. Able to use min gross grasp; AROM includes shoulder ✓ 60°, elbow ✓ 30°; 1 finger subluxation noted. Min edema noted in hand.

Treatment Plan

1. Pt oriented x 3 in 1 wk.
2. Pt able to sit ↔ supine c̄ min (A) in 1 wk.
3. Pt ↑ activity tolerance to 25 min @ bedside in 1 wk.
4. Pt able to complete basic grooming skills in 1 wk.
5. Pt will show ↑'d AROM @ (R) sh to 85°.

Outline 4 tx sessions:

❏ Make sure to consider pt's physical and cognitive status, activity tolerance, and goals.
❏ Include daily PROM of (R) UE.

The pt has a Dx of (R) THR with a hx of severe RA (posterior approach). Her therapy is scheduled 30 minutes q.d. for 3 days in acute care hospital. She lives in a nursing home. Her discharge plan is to return to the nursing home. The pt has multiple joint deformities, including min functioning shoulder joints and nonfunctioning fingers.

A. Diagnosis: THR

❑ Look up as total hip arthroplasty: Surgical replacement of head and neck of the femur. Process that cements a self-curing acrylic resin to adhere a plastic acetabular cup to the pelvis and a metal prosthetic femoral head to the hollowed-out femur.
❑ Postoperative precautions (posterior approach): Avoid hip flexion past 70°–80° for first 2 months to allow soft tissue to heal after surgery. No passive range of motion of hip. Ambulation promoted quickly (full weight-bearing). ADL training to maintain hip precautions.

B. Phase of recovery:

❑ acute because of precautions

C. Facility considerations:

❑ patient seen 30 minutes each day for 2 weeks

D. Other significant areas:

❑ Patient lives in a nursing home and discharge plans are to return to the nursing home.
❑ Severe RA: A systemic disease characterized by remissions and exacerbations that vary in severity and timing among people. Symptoms involve pain, stiffness, and limited movement in joints, malaise, fatigue, wasting of muscles around joints, and anemia. After an exacerbation, joints are left progressively deformed. Treatment approach is prevention of joint deformity and pain for as long as possible. Excess joint play is due to loosened ligaments and joint capsules and contracture of muscles and other connective tissue.

Occupational Therapy Evaluation Summary

Cognitive Status: Pt's cog status is WFL, including communication and problem solving.

UE Status: AROM significantly limited @ shoulders, elbows, and hands. Shoulder ✓ 85° (R), elbow / at −40° (B). Pt shows min gross grasp c̄ (R) hand fingers only (not thumb). (L) hand shows no grasp ability. Muscle testing not completed 2° to Dx.

Gross Motor: Pt requires mod (A) to roll → (L) 2° to pain. Rolling → (R) requires min (A). Sit ↔ supine requires max (A). Transfers are mod (A) 2° to ↓'d WB on (R) LE. Sitting balance f+.

ADL Status: Dependent for self-feeding, UE and LE dressing, and basic grooming.

Treatment Plan

1. Pt able to feed self c̄ adaptive equipment in 1 wk.
2. Pt able to perform transfers c̄ min (A) in 1 wk.
3. Pt able to roll (R) and (L) c̄ SBA in 1 wk.
4. Pt able to perform basic grooming tasks c̄ adaptive equipment in 1 wk.

Outline 4 tx sessions:

❏ Make sure to consider physical limitations and be specific on adaptive equipment recommendations.

Tom is an 82 y/o M in an ICU (see Figure 1.4).

Referral reads

- ❏ Dx: L CVA.
- ❏ Evaluate and treat.

Medical chart information

- ❏ R parietal CVA s/p 2 days
- ❏ DM
- ❏ MI s/p 2 months
- ❏ Patient lives with wife and required her assistance for ADL prior to admit.

Figure 1.4   Tom

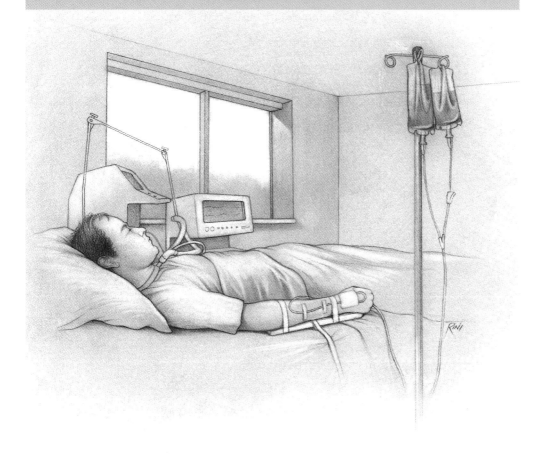

Medications

❏ Heparin
❏ Procardia®
❏ Humulin® insulin NPH (neutral protamine hagedorn—long-acting)

When you approach Tom, he is in bed supine with an IV in his right arm, a urinary catheter, and three leads from an ECG monitor on his chest for tracking his heart condition. He appears very tired and is slow to respond to your questions. Treatment should be kept short because of his medical condition.

Occupational Therapy Evaluation Summary

Cognitive Status: Pt oriented × 2, shows severe (R) visual neglect, able to understand directions and explanations, responds c̄ short statements 2° to fatigue. Able to follow 1- and 3-step commands. Pt alert for two 20-min periods.

(L) UE Status: PROM WFL; coordination and sensation intact; strength F.

Gross Motor: Pt able to roll R ↔ L c̄ mod (A); low level activity tolerance of 10 min; able to recover in 5 min. Head control fair-.

Treatment Plan

1. Pt able to tolerate low-level activities for 25 min in 1 wk.
2. ↑ head control to WFL in 1 wk.
3. Pt able to compensate for visual neglect c̄ physical cues in 1 wk.
5. ↓ edema in (L) hadn to min in 1 wk.

Outline 4 tx sessions:

❏ Provide PROM to (L) UE in each session.
❏ Explain how you would cue pt to compensate for his visual neglect.

Sara is a 23 y/o F currently in an acute care facility with the possibility of going to a rehabilitation unit.

Referral reads

❏ Dx: (L) UE below-elbow amputee.
❏ Eval the potential for UE prosthesis.

Medical chart information

❏ (L) UE below-elbow amputee s/p 1 wk.
❏ No other significant medical hx.

Sara was involved in a car accident. She enjoys horseback riding, reading, and playing various sports. She works as a data processor. She is currently taking various courses at the community college, with no major declared.

❏ What other service could you contact to determine the financial and insurance information you need to help determine your recommendations? What information do you need to know?

Occupational Therapy Evaluation Summary

Cognitive Status: Intact for problem-solving and safety.

ADL Status: Basic grooming skills intact, including makeup, UE dressing WFL, LE dressing requires mod (A); home living tasks require mod (A) 2° to ↓'d (B) UE functioning.

UE Status: (R) UE AROM is WFL; strength G; gross- and fine-motor coordination intact. Sensation intact. (L) UE: elbow/shoulder AROM is WFL; strength F+. Gross-motor coordination intact @ shoulder and elbow. Pt shows ↑'d sensitivity @ surgery site. Pt shows mod edema below elbow. Wound site is closed c̄ sutures in place.

Gross Motor: Transfers, bed mobility, and ambulation intact.

Treatment Plan

1. Pt able to complete skin care self-inspection in 1 wk.
2. Pt independent c̄ UE dressing in 1 wk.
3. ↑ (L) UE strength to N @ shoulder and elbow in 1 wk.
4. Pt able to complete cooking and cleaning activities independently in 1 wk.

Outline 4 tx sessions:

❑ Include ↓'ing wound sensitivity techniques.
❑ Include training and *explanation* for use of a stump sock or ACE bandage.
❑ Explain techniques for household activities using the (L) UE as an assist for functioning.

Nancy is a 32 y/o F. She is an outpatient referred to your clinic.

Referral reads

❏ Dx: RA.
❏ Eval for baseline information and provide education for arthritis care.

Medical chart information

❏ RA, onset 1 year ago.
❏ Nancy is a homemaker with two children, 7 and 4 years old. Her primary complaint is joint pain currently confined to her hands.

Medications

❏ Nonsteroidal antiinflammatory (NSAID).
❏ Prednisone injection to (L) shoulder 2 days ago.

Occupational Therapy Evaluation Summary

UE Status: A/PROM WFL (B) for all joints; hands and wrists show nonstructural deviations. Strength F+ of (R) UE, G of (L) UE. Gross- and fine-motor coordination intact. Sensation intact (B).

Cognitive Status: WFL for all areas including problem solving and safety.

Gross Motor: Ambulation, bed mobility, and gross-motor activities WFL. Pt reports she tolerates approx. 45 min–1 hr of activity.

Treatment Plan

1. Pt will demonstrate an understanding of energy conservation techniques in 1 wk.
2. Pt will eval and select adaptive equipment for ADL in 1 wk.
3. Pt will identify methods of adapting her DLS to ↓ the symptoms of her disease in 1 wk.
4. Pt will be able to identify and participate in activities that will ↓ the symptoms of RA in 1 wk.

Outline 3 (1 hr) tx sessions:

❑ Make sure to address all areas of the tx plan because Nancy will be d/c'd in 1 wk.
❑ Include HOs and activity suggestions.

Warren is a 68 y/o M on a rehabilitation unit to receive his prosthesis and gait training.

Referral reads

❑ Eval/tx for ADL status.

Medical chart information

❑ (R) BKA s/p 1 wk.
❑ IDDM.
❑ Cardiac arrhythmia.
❑ Questionable hx of ETOH abuse.

Medications

❑ Humulin® insulin NPH.
❑ Inderal®.
❑ Tylenol® #3 p.r.n.

In the interview, Warren indicates he is a retired high school coach. He swam every day up until 2 weeks before surgery, and he enjoys playing golf. Warren is complaining of pain in his (R) foot while he is sitting in his chair and says it is worse at night while he is sleeping.

Occupational Therapy Evaluation Summary

UE Status: AROM and strength WFL (B); sensation mod impair in (B) hands (sharp/dull and temperature).

Gross Motor: Static/dynamic sitting balance intact. Transfers w/c ↔ mat and bed SBA; w/c ↔ reg chair min (A); bed mobility independent. Transfers from floor mod (A); standing balance f, tolerance 5 min s̄ prosthesis. Pt shows min WB on (R) prosthesis during transfers and standing. W/c mobility independent.

Cognitive Status: Intact throughout.

ADL Status: Independent for grooming, UE and LE dressing; requires (A) to don/doff prosthesis.

Treatment Plan

1. Pt able to don/doff prosthesis independently in 1 wk.
2. Pt will show mod weight-bearing on (R) LE c̄ prosthesis in 1 wk.
3. Pt will be able to demonstrate skin self-inspection in 1 wk.
4. Pt able to tolerate standing activities c̄ prosthesis for 20 min in 1 wk.
5. Pt requires SBA for transfers floor ↔ w/c s̄ prosthesis in 1 wk.
6. Pt able to wrap stump independently in 1 wk.

Outline 4 tx sessions:

❏ Include an explanation of why he is feeling pain in his (R) foot. How would you explain his situation?
❏ Make activities purposeful and functional.
❏ Include HO for stump-wrapping technique.

Mary is a 42 y/o F in an acute care hospital.

Referral reads

- ❏ Dx: aneurysm.
- ❏ Eval and tx.

Medical chart information

- ❏ Aneurysm burst s/p 1 week; pt underwent clipping for 2 aneurysms s/p 1 wk; location involved cerebellum and (L) temporal lobe.
- ❏ CT of head indicates min edema. Lesions in (L) temporal lobe and cerebellum.

Mary was preparing dinner for her family. She indicated she had a headache earlier that evening to her husband. She told her husband she was feeling sick to her stomach and went to lie down. Her husband went to check on her about 45 minutes later and was unable to wake her. She was taken to the hospital and underwent evacuation for the hemorrhage, followed by a CT of the head. The following day, she underwent surgery for clipping of another aneurysm.

Medications

- ❏ Nimodipine for 21 days.
- ❏ Heparin.

Mary is in a regular w/c. She is alert and has her hands lying in her lap. You explain that you are an occupational therapy assistant and why she is here to see you. You ask Mary how she is feeling today and she does not reply. You then ask her to raise her arms up in the air. Mary looks away from you and grasps her hands together in her lap.

Occupational Therapy Evaluation Summary

Cognitive Status: Pt demonstrates mod receptive/expressive aphasia; she is able to verbally respond c̄ single-word responses. Unable to test direction-following 2° to physical status. Pt shows mod (R) visual neglect.

Physical Status: Sitting balance good; P/AROM of UEs WFL. Coordination of UE movements poor; pt has difficulty performing repetitive UE activities. Strength appears WFL; no subluxation noted; no edema noted. Fine-motor coordination severely impaired. Transfers w/c ↔ mat mod (A). Bed mobility mod (A).

ADL Status: Pt dependent for grooming, UE and LE dressing and bathing.

Treatment Plan

1. Pt able to perform basic grooming tasks c̄ setup in 1 wk.
2. Pt able to transfer w/c ↔ mat in 1 wk.
3. Pt able to don/doff shirt independently in 1 wk.
4. Pt able to complete simple (C) UE activities in 1 wk.

Outline 4 tx sessions:

❏ What technique would you use for explaining how to dress and complete grooming?
❏ Make sure to incorporate techniques to ↓ (R) visual neglect during activities and explain how you would accomplish this.

Beulah is a 79 y/o F. She is placed in a rehabilitation unit for physical and occupational therapy services.

Referral reads

- ❑ Dx: (R) hip fx c̄ THR.
- ❑ Evaluate and treat.

Medical chart information

- ❑ Hx of Parkinson's disease.
- ❑ UTI.
- ❑ THR (R), 2 days s/p.
- ❑ (B) WBAT.
- ❑ Patient to be poseyed at all times.
- ❑ Patient lives with her daughter, Carol. She required constant supervision, and Carol helped her c̄ her self-care activities.

Medications

- ❑ Parlodel®.
- ❑ Macrodantin®.
- ❑ Tylenol® #3 p.r.n.
- ❑ Guidelines for total hip precautions.

As you approach Beulah, she is in a wheelchair with a waist posey, and she is carrying a towel. She is talking very quietly to herself. The initial interview is as follows:

Thelma (Therapist): "Hi, Beulah, my name is Thelma. I am an occupational therapist. Your doctor asked me to see you to help you get back on your feet."
Beulah: "Nice to meet you, Thelma. Thanks for coming over. Would you like something to eat?"
Thelma: "No, thank you. Beulah, do you know where you are?"
Beulah: "Why, yes. I am at home with my mother and father. This is my baby, Tami. Isn't she sweet?"
Thelma: "Beulah, you are in the hospital right now. Do you live alone?"
Beulah: "Yes, I've lived alone all my life. My good plates are gone. Someone must have stolen them." (Beulah begins to cry.)
(Thelma gets some bright-colored pegs and a bucket and puts them on a table in front of Beulah.)
Thelma: "Can you put these pegs in this bucket for me, please?"

Beulah: "Sure I can." (Beulah tries to reach up for the pegs; her movements are slow and appear rigid. She is unable to complete putting the pegs in the bucket without physical and verbal cues.)

❏ What other hospital service could you contact to get a history and living situation on Beulah, and what kind of information do you need?

Outline 4 tx sessions:

❏ Include activities to ↑ general UE ROM and ↓ fear of movement.
❏ Because of her fear of movement and cognitive status, it is best to make all activities concrete, functional, and purposeful.

Treatment Plan

1. Pt demonstrate functional transfers c̄ SBA in 1 week.
2. ↑ pt standing balance to good.
3. ↑ pt functional mobility to SBA.
4. Provide family c̄(3) activities pt can participate in @ home.

References

American Occupational Therapy Association. (1993). Occupational therapy roles. *American Journal of Occupational Therapy, 43,* 1087–1099.

American Occupational Therapy Association. (1994). Uniform terminology for occupational therapy (3rd ed.). *American Journal of Occupational Therapy, 48,* 1047–1054.

DeLisa, J. A., Martin, G. M., & Currie, D. M. (1988). Rehabilitation medicine: Past, present, and future. In J.A. DeLisa (Ed.). *Rehabilitation medicine: Principles and practice* (pp. 7–8) Philadelphia: Lippincott.

Hopkins, H. L., & Smith, H. D. (Eds.). (1983). *Willard and Spackman's occupational therapy* (6th ed.). Philadelphia: Lippincott.

National Case Management Task Force Steering Committee. (1991, pamphlet). *Work summary and survey of case management toward medical case manager certification.* Little Rock, AK: Systematic.

National Therapeutic Recreation Society. (1992). *Therapeutic recreation: A comprehensive approach to a continuum of care.* Alexandria, VA: Author.

Puckett, R. P., & Miller, B. B. (1988). *Food service manual for health care institutions.* Chicago: American Hospital Publishing.

Weed, L. L. (1971). *Medical records, medical education, and patient care.* Cleveland, OH: Press of Case Western Reserve University.

Bibliography

Christiansen, C., & Baum, C. (1991). *Occupational therapy: Overcoming human performance deficits.* Thorofare, NJ: Slack.

Ryan, S. (Ed). (1993a). *The certified occupational therapy assistant: Principles, concepts, and techniques* (2nd ed.). Thorofare, NJ: Slack.

Ryan, S. (1993b). *Practice issues in occupational therapy intraprofessional team building.* Thorofare, NJ: Slack.

CHAPTER 2

Treatment Planning Process

Objectives

After completing the exercises in this chapter, the student should be able to

❏ identify guidelines for assisting the OTR in setting up a treatment plan

❏ collaborate with the OTR in writing objective goals with respect to the patient's current status

❏ select appropriate activities that correspond to the treatment goals, based on activity analysis

❏ describe occupational therapy treatment techniques that address a patient's physical or cognitive symptoms

❏ identify patient and professional behaviors that interfere with communication

❏ identify effective communication characteristics.

Introduction

Larry is in his third week of clinical affiliation training at an acute care hospital with a 10-bed rehabilitation unit. He has been assigned a couple of patients and is feeling good about the therapy activities he is providing. He is beginning to feel like a professional therapist. His supervisor assigned a new patient, George, to his caseload.

CASE STUDY: George

George had a stroke 5 days ago. The OT's evaluation indicated that he could not roll over or sit up. He had problems understanding instructions, his right side was flaccid, and he was severely neglecting the right side of his body. Larry realized that these were the only areas evaluated now because George's endurance was still very low. There were a lot of things unknown about George's deficits. The social worker's report indicates that the family will take him home, and there would be no other discharge considerations. George seemed so far away from achieving that plan or for any self-care aspects of therapy.

The OT's treatment plan included goals of ↑'ing bed mobility, sitting balance, and ↑'ing self-grooming skills, and facilitating function of his (R) UE. His supervisor asked him to outline 3 tx sessions based on the goals.

Larry decided to get a candy bar. On his way to the cafeteria, he started thinking about George. "Where do I start? There are so many problem areas. He cannot understand anything, he cannot sit, stand, or use his (R) arm, and he cannot see half of his world. What are some of his other deficits we cannot even see yet? How can he possibly go home c̄ his family? Why did my supervisor give me this patient? I am not ready for this, and she knows it."

This is a common situation faced by developing therapists. It seems that as soon as a student begins feeling comfortable with his or her skills, he or she is presented with a new challenge. It is the purpose of the clinical affiliation and the responsibility of the supervisor to continue challenging the student toward professional independence. The process can be uncomfortable; however, there are several things the student can do to ease the learning process. The student can learn about and contribute to the treatment planning process; he or she can use his or her school references and communicate with his or her supervisor. He or she cannot expect the supervisor to provide all the answers to every question, but he or she can foster professional communication to assist in problem solving.

Section I   Setting Up Treatment Plans

The OTR, after evaluating the patient, will have identified a problem or a set of problems that need to be addressed. In addition, the OTR establishes the patient's condition based on the diagnosis, chart review, age, prognosis, and past living situation, as well as future living arrangements, if known. As a result of the evaluation, the OTR also addresses the current status of the patient. This comes from objective testing, as well as information gathered from others, including other disciplines or the patients' families or significant others. The COTA may have contributed to this by screening or interviewing the patient or assisting with giving standardized tests under supervision.

Based on the initial evaluation, long-term and short-term goals are established. The steps needed to achieve these goals become the treatment plan. Goal setting involves using functional activities that can be measured.

How do the supervising therapist and OTA student establish what activities should be used in achieving the goals? The process used in choosing the appropriate activities to accomplish the goals is called *activity analysis*. This is an integral part of treatment planning. Experienced therapists automatically analyze activities, based on past experiences, in setting goals. Students need to spend some time in analyzing activities. Many types of activity analysis exist. Next we will discuss the components that many have in common (Ryan, 1993, p. 227).

One of the areas in the activity analysis process with which students have difficulty is adapting and grading the activities. How do you change an activity, and how can you make it easier or more challenging for the patient? *Adapting* or *modifying* an activity means to change the way an activity is done. Adaptation incorporates allowing the patient to perform at his or her level of functioning (Ryan, 1993, p. 226). For example, a patient with a CVA and use of only one upper extremity needs to learn one-handed techniques to don a shirt. *Grading* means to progress from simple to complex (Ryan, 1993, p. 226). The process of donning the shirt may be progressing from donning the shirt in 3 minutes to donning it in 1 minute. Also, the level of assistance needed could be expected to decrease—for example, from total assistance to independent.

Treatment plans should be reviewed and changed according to the patient's progress. In actual treatment situations, the COTA usually works with the patient after the OTR has finished the evaluation and turns the patient over to the COTA. The COTA may have participated in the evaluation process, but often the COTA has not seen the patient. During the affiliation, the OTR should involve the OTA student with the evaluation process as much as possible. Scheduled meetings with the OTR are necessary. The OTA student should be aware of the goals and the need to follow the prescribed plan. An important part of the OTA student's contribution to the treatment plan is to notice any changes in the performance of the patient and to report this change to the supervising therapist. For example, a patient may be able to complete an activity in the expected time without difficulties and has thus achieved a goal. This should be noted, and the supervising therapist informed. Noting changes in the performance of a patient and recognizing the need to change the treatment plan accordingly often are difficult for students. Sometimes the same activities are used repeatedly when the patient needs to progress to a more challenging task. With ever-shortening hospital and rehabilitation stays, it is crucial to allow the patient to progress as efficiently as possible.

Being familiar with the components of activity analysis and knowing how to adapt and grade activities to achieve goals are closely connected to the treatment planning process. The process of setting up a treatment plan can be broken down into four sections or questions that identify where the patient is, the patient's current status, the patient's goals, and therapeutic methods to reach those goals. Exploring these areas allows the therapist to combine these facts and formulate a plan that facilitates independence while taking into consideration the facility limitations, the patient's abilities and goals, and the discharge plans. This is the process an OTR goes through, and COTAs may need to participate. The process is designed to change the treatment plan as the patient progresses.

Where Is the Patient?

Asking "where is the patient" pertains to the patient's current situation. Information can include the patient's current diagnosis, past medical history, and age, all of which help determine life-cycle status and current medical precautions. It also can include the patient's previous or current living situation.

The facility situation and prognosis are valuable considerations when assessing the patient's situation. The combination of this information provides input to past and current physical and cognitive limitations or assets.

What Is the Patient's Current Status?

The current status describes the patient's strengths and weaknesses. This information is gathered from the objective testing during an occupational therapy evaluation and from objective reports from other disciplines. Gathering and reviewing objective test information use basic skills that can be enhanced to accomplish goals related to the entire treatment plan.

What Are the Patient's Goals?

The patient's goals are the major focus of this question. However, other areas also should be considered: family input, discharge placement, and future therapeutic intervention options.

For example, a patient who has suffered a CVA and is at an acute care hospital, with an average length of stay of 3 days, may have a goal of preparing for short-term rehabilitation that has a length of stay from 6 to 8 weeks. Thus, the patient's goal to walk may be unrealistic during the acute hospital stay.

What Therapeutic Methods Are Needed to Reach the Goals?

The therapist identifies the major skills that the patient will need to reach the stated goals. These skills become the long-term goals of the treatment plan. The therapist then identifies the specific skills that the patient will need to accomplish long-term goals. These skills become the short-term goals of the treatment plan. The therapist then reexplores the theory options that fit the situation and outlines therapy activities that address the short-term goals.

Finally, the therapist should consider the importance of requesting referrals from other disciplines (Day, 1973; Hemphill, 1982; Pedretti, 1985). Today's health care environment requires efficient rehabilitation care. Obtaining information from various disciplines assists in devising a complete therapy plan in an efficient and timely manner. Other disciplines add different perspectives to an individual's physical and mental status that can be an asset to the recovery process and the total treatment plan. This interaction enables the entire team to function together toward mutual goals for the patient's recovery process.

Practical Application

Complete exercises 2:1–2:5. These exercises are designed to illustrate how a treatment plan varies according to information that is gathered.

Section II   Objectives for Effective Goal Writing

The therapy plan outlines the focus areas of treatment and helps the therapist refine the type of theoretical approach used to provide therapy intervention. The therapist does not document the entire therapy plan. The treatment process is tracked through documentation of subjective, objective, assessment, and plan information. This is meant to be a summary or outline of the therapy plan that has been developed. The therapeutic plan consists of long- and short-term goals. These goals should always be reflected in a functional aspect relating to the patient's or family members' abilities.

The purpose of treatment goals is to enhance understanding of the value of treatment by third party payers, other health care providers, and consumers (Kuntavanish, 1987). *Consumers* refers to the patient's family members who are involved in the occupational therapy process.

A goal should be descriptive of the focus of treatment. It should address the functional ability of the patient or family member that the treatment plan is attempting to change, and it should be measurable. A goal can be broken into three components: *verbs*, the *functional area of focus*, and the *measurable end point*. (Figure 2.1 provides examples of these.)

Verbs

Verbs describe the desirable action that the treatment plan is attempting to achieve. They relate to actions performed by the patient or family member, not the therapist. This part of the goal describes the change occupational therapy treatment is expected to produce.

Functional Area of Focus

The *functional area of focus* refers to the skills or activities the treatment plan addresses. These components, which relate to improving function while receiving appropriate therapeutic intervention techniques, can be passive or active.

Figure 2.1 Functional areas of focus, verbs, and measurable end points

VERB	FUNCTIONAL AREA OF FOCUS	MEASURABLE END-POINT
demonstrate	PROM	Goniometer measurement
strengthen	AROM	Dynamometer
increase	A/AROM	Standardized tests
decrease	hand grip household mobility	Achieved a functional act: reach in refrigerator, tolerate w/c positioning
recall achieve perform	UE dressing LE dressing	Reflects the amount of (A) required to complete tasks: verbal cues, min, mod, max (A)
identify	THR precautions muscle tone	Muscle-testing grading system
list interpret recall apply use	any specific muscle any specific joint pivot transfers standing tolerance sitting balance	Minutes or time # of repetitions
state classify construct describe	w/c mobility self-feeding physical endurance strength	Any method the pt is able to show understanding verbally, in writing, on computer

Measurable End Point

The *measurable end point* indicates the specific desired objective being addressed in the treatment plan. This section also can include the functional aspect of the treatment process.

There are several methods that can be used to document the measurable end point. The chosen method should be as objective as possible and should be used throughout the treatment process.

For example, if the method of measurement for improving upper-extremity endurance is the number of exercise repetitions a patient is able to perform during therapy, it should not change to time-related measures.

The following case study of Bob illustrates the link between the treatment planning process and the development of short- and long-term goals.

Bob has a diagnosis of CVA. His evaluation and tx plan were to be completed within 24 hours. His occupational therapy evaluation results are listed below:

O: Upper extremity status:

(L) UE ROM and strength are WFL.
(R) UE shows flaccid tone throughout; he has no subluxation, and PROM is WFL; sensation was not tested.

Cognitive status:

Pt able to follow and understand directions. He asks appropriate questions related to recovery. He shows poor ability to sequence skills for dressing.

Transfer status:

Pt requires mod A × 1 for stand-pivot transfers w/c ↔ mat.

Self-care:

Pt dependent for LE dressing. He requires max A for UE dressing 2° to poor sequencing skills.

A: Strengths:
❏ left side UE and LE are strong and show AROM WFL
❏ eager and motivated to work on recovery
❏ able to understand and follow directions

Weaknesses:
❏ unable to sequence steps for dressing tasks
❏ right UE flaccid and PROM WFL, no subluxation
❏ unable to completely bear weight on (R)LE

Discharge destination:
❏ home c̄ wife and 18 y/o daughter
❏ wife does not work outside the home

Major skills needed:
❏ Transfers ↔ commode, tub, and regular chairs
❏ Dressing skills ↔ UE and LE
❏ Maintain and/or facilitate (R) UE status

Figure 2.2 Bob's case study chart

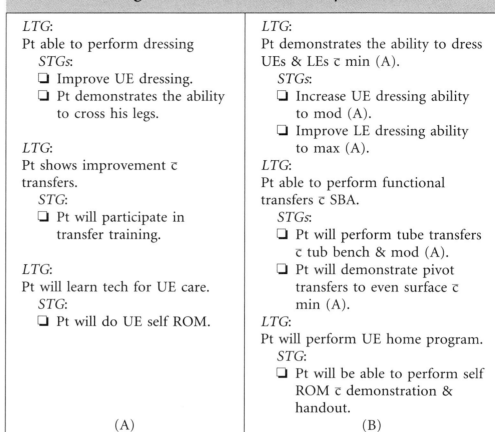

LTG:
Pt able to perform dressing
  STGs:
    ❏ Improve UE dressing.
    ❏ Pt demonstrates the ability
      to cross his legs.

LTG:
Pt shows improvement c̄
transfers.
  STG:
    ❏ Pt will participate in
      transfer training.

LTG:
Pt will learn tech for UE care.
  STG:
    ❏ Pt will do UE self ROM.

(A)

LTG:
Pt demonstrates the ability to dress
UEs & LEs c̄ min (A).
  STGs:
    ❏ Increase UE dressing ability
      to mod (A).
    ❏ Improve LE dressing ability
      to max (A).
LTG:
Pt able to perform functional
transfers c̄ SBA.
  STGs:
    ❏ Pt will perform tube transfers
      c̄ tub bench & mod (A).
    ❏ Pt will demonstrate pivot
      transfers to even surface c̄
      min (A).
LTG:
Pt will perform UE home program.
  STG:
    ❏ Pt will be able to perform self
      ROM c̄ demonstration &
      handout.

(B)

In Figure 2.2, Section A represents examples of poor goal writing. The goals are not consistently stated in terms of the patient performing a functional task. They also do not document a measurable end point. It would be difficult to visualize the patient's current abilities or his projected skill development from this treatment plan. However, Section B describes functional projections for the long-term goals and specific task development for each short-term goal. A person reading this treatment plan can clearly see the functional progression to recovery.

Practical Application

Complete exercises 2:6–2:13. These are designed to be a continuation of the treatment planning process and provide goal-writing opportunities.

Sarah is completing her sixth week of clinical affiliation. She has a full caseload and is doing her treatment planning and direct care without much supervision. Sarah is sitting down to complete her weekly notes on the progress and status of each of her patients. As she is organizing her work, she thinks about the different personalities of each of her patients and how they respond to the therapy process.

- ❑ Debbie is a registered nurse (RN) who suffered a severe stroke. She has difficulty sitting up and eating. Her left side is nonfunctional, and her communication and speech comprehension are poor. However, Debbie is the most motivated, energetic patient on Sarah's caseload. She will try anything, and she is the type of patient who will show you something new that she learned on her own.

- ❑ Derek is an outpatient who broke his wrist. When the cast was removed, he had limited movement and strength in his nondominant hand and wrist. Every therapy session, Derek emphasizes everything he cannot do. He has quit work, and his wife helps him with dressing and with his hygiene needs. Sarah has made several suggestions to both Derek and his wife that would allow him to return to a more normal daily routine; however, they always convey frustrating descriptions relating to his inability to do anything for himself.

- ❑ Bob suffered a stroke recently. He had a slight decrease of functional use of his right side. Communication is intact, and he has a few other minor deficits. Sarah taught Bob to propel his wheelchair the first day of therapy. Bob is extremely grateful. Every chance he gets, he expresses his gratitude for her help and knowledge.

- ❑ Martha had a hip replacement after falling down a flight of stairs. She had a few other bruises and several cracked ribs. It has been a week, and she is walking around the kitchen, cooking, going on outings with recreational therapy, and is preparing to go home. However, she does not see any progress with her recovery pattern. Her mood and behavior are the same as the first day Sarah saw her. Regardless of what Sarah says regarding Martha's progress, Martha feels she is not recovering because she is still using a walker.

- ❑ John was hit by a car and broke his clavicle and left femur. John cannot be classified as motivated or unmotivated—he just does what he is asked to do. He really does not offer any of his own opinions of the therapeutic process. John is always making jokes and often is the highlight of the therapy clinic. However, yesterday, Sarah said her usual "Good morning, John, how are you?" and John burst into tears.

Patient Reaction to Health Care

There are many reasons why patients react differently to the health care process. First, the hospital or rehabilitation process has a definite impact on the patient. In addition, the patient's illness causes a great deal of anxiety. The patient also may be concerned about role obligations, including family responsibilities, financial issues, and deterioration of friendships (DiMatteo, 1991).

The patient may experience a loss of control, independence, and privacy. DiMatteo (1991) has described the expected hospital patient role as "cooperative, pleasant, and quiet unless there is an emergency." This expectation has been established by the health care system. Health care professionals generally must have heavy caseloads in order to meet cost-effective productivity expectations. They also tend to depersonalize patients' situations. This is a defense mechanism to protect themselves from the discomfort that may occur from working with patients on a personal level. These factors may lead caregivers to treat all patients the same, in a quick and efficient manner, rather than on an individual basis.

For example, suppose a nurse has four patients to work with during a shift. Everyone gets a bed bath between 7:00 A.M. and 8:00 A.M. If a patient needs assistance in using the bathroom, he or she may have to wait for help because the nurse is passing out medications to all the patients. As a result, the patient assigned to this nurse has lost his or her ability to control when to use the bathroom or take a bath. These are not characteristics of poor nursing care; they are characteristics of the health care system.

Different patients react to these situations in different ways. Loss of control can cause anxiety because the patient may develop inadequate expectations or confusion. Feeling helpless or being powerless also can cause anxiety or depression. Some patients react angrily to these situations. Others react with denial, and still others react by developing good patient behavior that can lead to feeling helpless.

Looking at the research that has explored the patients' rationale for accessing health care services can help to explain how and why patients react differently to health care and rehabilitation. The same information can give professional insight into why an individual responds or does not respond to therapeutic treatment.

Some individuals are more likely to notice and attend to a symptom or body disorder than others (Mandler & Kahn, 1960). There are also individuals who will continue with their normal daily routine regardless of any pain or discomfort. In addition, there are individuals who are unable to function with any type of abnormality. A person's self-interpretation of his or her illness can be related to his or her current situation, stress level, or mood. Any of these factors may indicate to an individual that he or she can attend to the current situation or that other factors in his or her life may appear to be more important.

Patients also interpret symptoms based on several other factors. Prior experience or expectations can greatly influence how a person will react to a health problem. A woman who cared for her mother after a stroke during the last few months of the mother's life, may react differently after she herself suffers a stroke than a woman who has had no contact with a stroke victim.

The interpretation of the seriousness of an illness varies from individual to individual. A young girl with dreams of becoming a model may determine that a facial scar is more important to correct than visual perception and cognitive deficits, all of which have been the result of a car accident.

Finally, what the illness represents to an individual determines how he or she will react. Will the illness label the individual? What are the consequences of the illness?

Are there lifestyle changes or is there a long-term rehabilitation process? What does the individual perceive as the cause of the illness? What is the person's interpretation of the duration and cure for the illness (Lau & Hartman, 1983; Nerenz & Leventhal, 1983)?

An individual's interpretation of the use of the health care system and of rehabilitation can determine behavior traits. In addition, age and gender can cause different reactions to therapy. Men may look at illness and rehabilitation as a weakness. Older adults may be more receptive to illness because it is expected at their stage of life. A person's values, lifestyle, norms, and cultural interpretations also influence the way he or she will seek and respond to rehabilitation or health care in general (McKinlay, 1972).

Finally, after reviewing these complex issues that influence a patient's reaction to the therapy process, therapists should remember that it is possible that the individual may not have any of these reactions. The patient may just be tired, sick, and confused.

The principles and theories of occupational therapy specifically address the losses and frustrations that patients experience during a recovery process. The occupational therapy treatment plan that increases independence at any level can restore an individual's sense of control and self-sufficiency. The therapist should keep these patient reactions to health care in mind when providing treatment. This is essential for maintaining a working relationship with the person. In a busy clinic or hectic rehabilitation center, a therapist may unknowingly be contributing to the problems that cause a negative patient reaction rather than providing methods to relieve these difficult situations. This reinforces the need to consider the patient's goals for the therapy process. The therapist should make every effort to help the patient understand the current situation by explaining it at a level that can be accepted. Patients should be provided with opportunities to make choices whenever possible.

Considering the preceding factors, a therapist can have a difficult time providing the patient with a treatment plan and therapy intervention. Obtaining a patient's complete history can provide some insight into an individual's reaction to his or her current situation. However, it is impossible to learn everything about a person's past experiences, values, and lifestyle. The primary tool a therapist must rely on for ensuring effective patient interaction, regardless of these factors, is communication.

Communication Parameters

Communication is an extremely effective medium for assisting a patient through any therapy process. A professional with good communication skills will be able to develop a rapport with most people, regardless of the patients' physical and cognitive deficits. Developing a good rapport helps ensure that the patient will follow the recommendations provided by the professional.

However, several factors interfere with good communication. Poor listening skills are a deterrent. The occupational therapist may be very comfortable planning and providing effective methods of implementing treatment, but he or she may discontinue listening to what is important to the patient.

Being aware of nonverbal communication that conflicts with the patient's comments is an important listening skill. Nonverbal communication includes the patient's eye contact, facial expression, tone of voice, touch, and general body language, such as posture and limb movements. These signals may serve as a cue for the therapist to consider more options for gathering information. However, this is difficult to interpret when working with individuals who are physically or cognitively limited.

Listening also includes paying attention to families, friends, and other professionals. For example, suppose a young man is being seen by a therapist. During an initial family education process for his parents and sisters, he asks the therapist to provide information to a male friend. The therapist suggests that the friend attend the family meeting. Very shortly and quietly, the patient says, "Okay." He breaks eye contact and moves out of the room. On further investigation by the therapist, she discovers the patient and friend have a homosexual relationship. The therapist receives a release to be able to provide the friend with information, and conducts a separate education session. Effective use of verbal and nonverbal communication allows the patient and therapist to build a positive working relationship.

A major characteristic of effective verbal communication includes being polite. A therapist should introduce himself or herself. If working with a patient with cognitive or memory problems, introductions should take place daily to ensure recognition by the patient. Exchanging pleasant words and making eye contact with the patient are both important. The therapist should be in the patient's visual range (DiMatteo & DiNicola, 1982).

A therapist should also be aware of his or her use of nonverbal communication gestures. Patients often scrutinize medical professionals' behavior to discover clues about their condition or about what to expect. For example, a patient confided in her therapist that she was going crazy. The patient said she heard voices in her room and sometimes people grabbed her. The woman said, "I never see them, but I hear them. I can't sleep because I am afraid to close my eyes." The patient suffered from a severe right-sided visual neglect. The therapist discovered the incidents were related to the night nurses who turned the patient in bed and to a technician who came to draw the patient's blood. All of them were unaware of the severity of her visual deficit.

Another major characteristic of effective patient communication is empathy. As previously stated, it is impossible for a therapist to know all the influences and life experiences that affect an individual's behavior during the therapy process. However, empathetic therapists can help the patient overcome issues related to health care services. Carl Rogers has defined empathy as,

> A process that involves being sensitive to another individual's changing feelings and "connecting" emotionally to that other person. Empathy involves a process of "living for a line in the other person's life," entering his or her private perceptual world, and seeing events through his or her eyes. Empathy involves avoiding judgments about what the other is feeling and instead trying to understand fully those feelings from the person's perspective (as quoted in DiMatteo, 1991, p. 229).

Empathy takes practice. Being nonjudgmental of another's values is not always easy. However, effective use of empathy can enhance the therapeutic process because patients feel understood and feel that their concerns have been addressed. Patients also feel that they have had an active role in the decisions related to the treatment plan. These factors build a positive therapeutic relationship that can ensure successful follow-through with treatment recommendations.

Keeping Open the Lines of Communication (OTR/COTA)

OTA students have shorter affiliations than OT students. This means that the amount of time to get acquainted with a center is less. OTA students often feel uncertain of their ability to participate in the treatment planning and their role in the profession. If faced with uncertainty of their ability, OTA students may say to a supervisor that they do not know a certain procedure. For example, a supervising OTR or COTA may ask, "Do you know how to perform a ROM test?" The student feels insecure about the level of competency and states, "No, I don't." In reality, the student has had the opportunity to practice ROM in the classroom setting but still feels unprepared. A better answer would be, "I had this in class and have practiced on another student, but I would like more hands-on experience." In this manner, both the supervising therapist and the OTA student can better team up on treatment planning. The COTA's role in treatment planning is to contribute to the process. This, at times, seems vague. Much depends on the setting, the state licensure, and third party payers.

Practical Application

Complete exercises 2:14–2:21. These exercises are designed to explore situations that require communication skills for patients and family members involved in the rehabilitation process. These situations were selected to practice empathy skills when working with patients in realistic settings.

**TREATMENT
PLANNING
PROCESS**

A. Where is Anne now?

Anne is an 87 y/o F with diagnosis of multiple fractures secondary to a fall. She has a fractured (R) tibia and fx (R) radius. Currently, she is in full leg and full arm casts. Anne has been living in a nursing home for the past 5 years. Her medical hx includes dementia and osteoporosis. Anne's precautions are nonweight bearing on (R) LE or (R) UE.

B. What is Anne's current status?

UE Status: (R)UE PROM at shoulder WFL, strength not formally tested 2° to cast and the patient's poor direction following. Finger and thumb show mod edema. Color of fingers and nail beds pink, (L) UE AROM — WFL; strength appears about fair throughout, but not formally tested. Coordination is moderately impaired.

Cognitive Status: Pt not oriented to time or place. She is confused and has difficulty following simple directions. She is able to complete simple automatic responses and tasks. The patient occasionally cries in tx, apparently 2° to confusion.

Transfers: Pt requires max (A) to transfer w/c ↔ mat. She is unable to monitor the current no weight-bearing status on her (R) LE.

Gross-Motor Skills: Rolling R ↔ L requires mod (A); sit ↔ supine requires max (A) (pt appears fearful to move).

Self-Care: Pt dependent for donning/doffing sweater. She requires min (A) to feed self with nondominant hand. Other bathing & dressing dependent.

C. What are Anne's goals?

Anne will be returning to the nursing home. Before the fall, Anne was able to feed herself, get in and out of bed c̄ SBA, and perform bed mobility independently.

D. How can Anne reach these goals?

1. Identify Anne's strengths and weaknesses.

Strengths

❑ (L) UE AROM and strength are functional.
❑ Discharge placement is defined.
❑ (L) LE is functional.

Weaknesses

❑ Cognitive status (confusion and fear).
❑ ↓'d mobility (bed and transfers).
❑ ↓'d self-feeding.

2. Identify the major skills Anne will need to enable her to reach her desired destination. (List long-range goals.)

❏ ↑ transfer ability; ↓ fear; and ↑ safety.
❏ ↑ self-feeding skills.
❏ ↑ bed mobility skills.

All these skills will assist the caregivers in caring for Anne.

3. What specific skills will you need to address in order to work toward the major skills listed previously? Why? (List short-term goals.)

   a. Weight-bearing on (L) LE only to maintain circulation in order to work toward transferring using (L) LE only.
   b. Trunk rotation activities in chair to ↓ fear of movement.
   c. Coordination activities c̄ (L) UE to work toward self-feeding.

4. Identify two specific activities per area addressed in Section 3. Justify each activity in relation to Anne's weaknesses. Explain how to upgrade each activity.

   a. Weight-bearing on (L) LE only to maintain circulation in order to work toward transferring using (L) LE only.

Activity One

Have Anne stand at a counter c̄ your foot under her (L) LE and have her separate silverware (to maintain NWB status).

Justification

Relates to weakness areas of confusion. Sorting silverware will help Anne organize her thoughts because it is a simple, concrete, familiar activity. This should also ↓ her fear of standing because she is concentrating on the activity of sorting silverware.

Activity also relates to Anne's weakness of ↓'d mobility because it will ↑ her balance on her (R) LE, which will lead to improving her transferring ability.

Upgrade

Have Anne do a 1-handed activity while standing at the counter on her (L) LE that encourages her to reach. Example: Fold towels or put dishes away.

Activity Two

Practice stand–pivot transfers to and from even surfaces. Example: w/c ↔ mat.

Justification

Relates to weakness areas of fear and ↓'d mobility by practicing movement in a controlled setting with physical assistance. (May want to use a transfer belt to provide further security for the therapist and patient.)

Upgrade

Practice transfers on uneven surfaces. Example: On regular chairs or in and out of bed.

b. Trunk rotation activities in chair to ↓ fear of movement.

Activity One

Have Anne sit in a regular chair c̄ arms at a table and help you fold towels c̄ 1 hand.

Justification

Activity works on weakness area of confusion and fear. Anne is in a supported position and encouraged to do a familiar activity that involves movement.

Upgrade

Have Anne sit in an armless chair or on the bed for doing simple ADLs.

Activity Two

Have Anne sit EOM and pick up pegs on her (L) side (using her [R] hand) and throw them away in a trash can on her (R) side. (Therapist sits in front of her during the activity, on a stool.)

Justification

Relates to ↓'d mobility, fear, and confusion. This is a simple, repetitive task that encourages trunk rotation.

Upgrade

Have Anne pick up pegs on an object that has her reach toward the floor to further ↑ trunk movement.

c. Coordinate activities c̄ (L) UE to work toward self-feeding.

Activity One

Play simple card game c̄ card holder; have Anne put the cards in the holder.

Justification

Relates to weakness areas of confusion, fear, and ↓'d self-feeding. Anne's independence and practice in playing a simple card game will address all of these areas.

Upgrade

Practice counting out coins and money c̄ 1 hand.

Activity Two

Practice self-feeding; start c̄ finger foods.

Justification

Relates to weakness areas of confusion and ↓'d self-feeding. Self-feeding is a familiar task, so it would address her confused state and practice will ↑ her independence at mealtimes.

Upgrade

Practice self-feeding c̄ a spoon. Example: Use scrambled eggs.

EXERCISE 2:2 Carol

A. Where is Carol now?

Carol is a 28 y/o WF with Dx uncontrolled DM. She is legally blind in both eyes and continues to diminish. (R) BKA 6 months prior to current admission. She is now admitted because of gangrene in (L) foot and ankle. She has been admitted to receive whirlpool tx to the (L)LE, IV antibiotic tx, and possible amputation of (L) ankle/foot if infection remains uncontrollable. General prognosis to save the (L) LE is poor.

B. What is Carol's current status?

Subjective Information: Carol reports that she feels she is getting more dependent on her mother every day, and she does not like it.

Transfers: Pt indep c̄ functional transfers using crutches and weight bearing on (L) LE. Tub transfers indep c̄ crutches and tub transfer bench.

Gross-Motor Mobility: Independent rolling (R) and (L). She requires min (A) sit ↔ supine.

Equipment: Pt has transfer tub bench, crutches, and exercise equipment for UE and LE activities.

UE Functioning: Pt's UE are WFL (B) for AROM; strength is good − (B). No sign edema or skin tears noted. UE sensation stereognosis generally intact; sharp/dull and temperature impaired (B). Proprioception intact (B). Pt's gross-motor coordination is WFL (B). Fine-motor coordination is impaired (B), which appears 2° to ↓'d sensation in fingertip region.

Self-Care Skills: Pt requires mod (A) for dressing 2° to poor ability to orient clothes and requires (A) for standing during LE dressing. Bathing skills independent. Grooming skills require setup.

C. What are Carol's goals?

Carol was an RN and living in her own apt until 1 yr ago. She moved in c̄ her mother when her health deteriorated and she had to quit work. She will be returning home c̄ her mother. Both Carol and her mother realize that Carol's care is becoming more difficult as time passes. Carol feels guilty that she is becoming totally dependent on her mother. Carol's primary concern is she does not want her mother to have to lift her. Both Carol and her mother feel their relationship has changed, and they do not have anything they can enjoy together anymore.

D. How can Carol reach her goals?

1. Identify Carol's strengths and weaknesses.

Strengths

- ❑ Carol has equipment that can assist her at home.
- ❑ Her upper-extremity strength, skin condition, and active range of motion are assets.
- ❑ She appears motivated to assist her mother as much as she can with her self-care.

Weaknesses

- ❑ Functional transfer status could change secondary to prognosis of left foot/ankle.
- ❑ Upper extremity sensation is impaired bilaterally.
- ❑ Decreased visual status.
- ❑ Deteriorating health, which interferes with the relationship with her mother.
- ❑ Decreased gross mobility skills (sit-to-supine).

2. Identify the major skills Carol will need to enable her to reach her desired destination. (List long-range goals.)

- ❑ Increased upper-extremity strength to compensate for her possible loss of lower-extremity functioning.
- ❑ Increased ability to compensate for her decreased vision with ADL exercises to improve independence.
- ❑ Improved gross-motor skills (through training).
- ❑ Ways to stimulate a positive relationship between her and her mother.

3. What specific skills will you need to address in order to work toward the major skills listed previously? (List short-term goals.)

- a. Increase bilateral upper-extremity strength to *good*.
- b. Carol will be able to dress herself with minimal assistance.
- c. Carol will be independent for bed mobility (sit-to-supine).
- d. Carol and her mother will identify two leisure activities they can share.

4. Identify two specific activities per area addressed in Section 3.

- ❑ Justify each activity in relation to Carol's weaknesses.
- ❑ Explain how you would upgrade each activity.

a. Increase bilateral upper-extremity strength to *good.*

Activity One

Justification

Upgrade

Activity Two

Justification

Upgrade

b. Carol will be able to dress herself with minimal assistance.

Activity One

Justification

Upgrade

Activity Two

Justification

Upgrade

c. Carol will be independent for bed mobility (sit-to-supine).

Activity One

Justification

Upgrade

Activity Two

Justification

Upgrade

d. Carol and her mother will identify two leisure activities they can share.

Activity One

Justification

Upgrade

Activity Two

Justification

Upgrade

A. Where is Kevin now?

Kevin is 22 y/o c̄ a Dx of spinal cord injury—incomplete T-6. Kevin's Hx includes falling off the roof of his family's home while cleaning gutters 1 yr ago. He progressed from an acute care rehab program 4 months ago and went home c̄ his family. Since Kevin has been home, he basically has been staying in his house and yard. When he goes out, his father helps him c̄ his equip and car transfers.

B. What is Kevin's current status?

UE Status: AROM is WFL. Strength is normal or above for his age.

Cognitive Status: Pt's cog status intact for following complex directions. Pt shows good judgment and safety awareness.

Transfers: Bed and toilet transfers indep. Car transfers mod (A) x 1. Community functional transfers require mod (A). Floor transfers dependent. Tub bench transfers indep.

W/C Mobility: Indep within facility and in room. Pt requires freq verbal cues and occasional (A) outside of facility.

Balance: Dynamic sitting balance fair. Pt able to reach objects in w/c about knee height safely. Static balance WFL. Standing balance not tested.

Bed Mobility: Rolling (R) and (L) indep. Sit ↔ supine indep.

Self-Care: Pt indep for bathing, dressing, and grooming.

Equipment: Pt has transfer tub bench, hand-held shower, standard w/c, and Jay cushion.

C. What are Kevin's goals?

Kevin would like to return to college in the fall. It is currently May, and he has been accepted into the accounting program at a nearby university. He is also concerned that his parents are never going to let him live on his own. Kevin has a girlfriend of 3 years, and he is worried that their relationship is not going well. She is currently attending the university where Kevin was accepted. Kevin would like to live in a dorm room with his peers.

D. How can Kevin reach his goals?

1. Identify Kevin's strengths and weaknesses.

Strengths

❏ upper-extremity strength and range of motion status
❏ cognitive status
❏ age
❏ basic ADL status
❏ motivation for appropriate independent living skills.

Weaknesses

❏ community functional transfers
❏ community wheelchair mobility
❏ dynamic sitting balance
❏ equipment issued not appropriate to maximize independence
  (e.g., standard wheelchair)
❏ relationship with his parents appears to foster his dependence.

2. Identify the major skills Kevin will need to be able to go back to college. (List long-range goals.)

❏ increased community mobility
❏ increased functional transfers
❏ increased general independence and self-confidence to allow Kevin's relationship with his parents to develop toward his goals
❏ situational coping skills that will assist Kevin with his transition back to school and his role in the relationship with his girlfriend.

3. What specific skills and equipment needs will you have to address in order to work toward the major skills listed previously? Why? (List short-term goals.)

   a. Increase Kevin's ability to perform wheelchair mobility on various surface grades and in community settings.
   b. Teach Kevin advanced transfer skills to include floor transfers, community bathroom transfers, and car transfers.
   c. Assist Kevin in identifying leisure interest skills or hobbies and teach relaxation methods.

4. Identify two specific activities per area addressed in Section 3.

❏ Justify each activity in relation to Kevin's weaknesses.
❏ Explain how you would upgrade each activity.

a. Increase Kevin's ability to perform wheelchair mobility on various surface grades and in community settings.

Activity One

Justification

Upgrade

Activity Two

Justification

Upgrade

b. Teach Kevin advanced transfer skills to include floor transfers, community bathroom transfers, and car transfers.

Activity One

Justification

Upgrade

Activity Two

Justification

Upgrade

c. Assist Kevin in identifying leisure interest skills or hobbies and teach relaxation methods.

Activity One

Justification

Upgrade

Activity Two

Justification

Upgrade

A. Where is Ethel now?

Ethel is 79 y/o c̄ a Dx of (l)THR. Her medical Hx includes broken (R) wrist 1984, hysterectomy 1984 that resulted in bladder leakage, high blood pressure, and continuous medications; arthritis of (L) knee, and scleroderma on (B)UE. Her precautions include WBAT, no hip ✓ past 90°, no adduction past neutral. She needs to maintain these precautions for 8 wks. She is medically stable and will be discharged in 2 wks.

B. What is Ethel's current status?

Cog Status: Intact for orientation and direction following.

UE Strength: (L) prox strength G-; distal G; (R) prox G-; elbow ✓, pronation/ supination G; wrist/fingers G-.

Transfers: Mod x 2 s̄ ambulation device. Ethel only tolerates min. weight on her (L) LE during transfer. She requires mod (A) x 1 c̄ walker for 10- to 15-foot distances.

Balance: Static/dynamic sitting balance good, pt able to take full challenges in upright position; reaching past knees not tested 2° to THR precautions.

Bed Mobility: Rolling → (R) indep, rolling → (L) indep. with c/o pain, sit ↔ supine mod. x 1.

UE Status: Pt shows bright, shiny skin on (R) hand and about ⅓ of distal forearms. Pt shows multiple bumps in forearm area. Sensation intact. Shoulders and elbows show WFL for AROM (B). (B) hand coordination shows mod ↓'d functioning 2° to poor ability to completely grasp items.

Self-Care Skills: UE dressing slow, but independent. Pt dependent for LE dressing 2° to pain and THR precautions. Pt currently dependent for household mobility and requires mod (A) for self-bathing 2° to THR precautions.

Equipment: Pt currently does not have equipment at home.

C. What are Ethel's goals?

Ethel lived at home with her husband prior to this injury. She was independent with her self-care and household responsibilities. Ethel's husband works 3 days a week with their son at a neighborhood store. The business relies on him being there, so he will not be at home with Ethel every day. Ethel wants to return home and be as little burden as possible to her husband.

D. How can Ethel reach her goals?

1. Identify Ethel's strengths and weaknesses.

Strengths

❏ cognitive status
❏ general mobility
❏ motivation to return home as independent as possible

Weaknesses

❏ decreased weight-bearing on LLE secondary to pain
❏ hand functioning
❏ decreased functional mobility
❏ lack of assistive equipment for home use
❏ decreased ADL skills secondary to hip precautions

2. Identify the major skills Ethel will need in order to reach her goals. (List long-range goals.)

❏ She will need to be independent with dressing and maintaining her THR precautions.
❏ She will need to be independent in household mobility.
❏ She will need to maintain THR precautions during bathing and dressing, which will require equipment to assist her.

3. What specific skills will you need to address in order to work toward the major skills listed previously? (List short-term goals.)

a. dressing and bathing LEs
b. household mobility skills using the walker
c. training to use ADL equipment safely

4. Identify two specific activities per area addressed in Section 3.

❏ Justify each activity in relation to Ethel's weaknesses.
❏ Explain how you would upgrade each activity.

a. Dressing and bathing LEs

Activity One

Justification

Upgrade

Activity Two

Justification

Upgrade

b. Household mobility skills using the walker.

Activity One

Justification

Upgrade

Activity Two

Justification

Upgrade

c. Train her to use ADL equipment safely.

Activity One

Justification

Upgrade

Activity Two

Justification

Upgrade

A. Where is Schoci now?

Schoci is a 53 y/o with a hx of (L) CVA s/p 2 weeks. She is a very small, thin woman originally from Korea. She does not speak English at all. Her nephew is available 2 ×'s per week as an interpreter for the next 2 weeks. She has just been transferred from the acute care floor to a rehabilitation unit for 6 to 8 weeks. There is no other significant medical hx. Schoci lives with her sister and her family. She took care of the three children, cleaned the house, and prepared the meals.

B. What is Schoci's current status?

Orientation: The pt is oriented to person and is able to recognize her relatives, nurses, and therapists. Pt not oriented to time or place.

(R) UE Status: UE shows flaccid tone throughout. Shoulder is subluxed ½ finger. Pt shows min edema in hand and shows facial expression of pain at end ranges of PROM. PROM of UE WFL. No AROM noted with facilitation at this time.

(L) UE Status: AROM-WFL, strength fair+, coordination intact. No significant edema or subluxation noted. Normal tone. Pt grip strength 15#.

Posture/Head Control: WFL actively; pt sits with head turned to the left.

Transfers: Mod x 1 and SBA of another for w/c ↔ mat table.

Balance: Static sitting balance fair. Pt able to sit EOM safely without any challenges, such as reaching or pushing on trunk. Dynamic sitting balance poor. Unable to take any challenges to balance. Standing balance poor; pt shows min weight-bearing on (L) LE during standing.

Bed Mobility: Sit ↔ supine mod (A); roll → (R) min (A); roll → (L) max (A).

Sensation: Unable to accurately assess secondary to communication status. Pt responded to light touch stimuli both (R) and (L) UEs, and (R) stereognosis appears absent. (L) stereognosis appears intact.

Perception: Pt shows min (R) neglect. Unable to test perception; however, it appears functional during clinical observations.

Communication: Limited to reliable yes/no responses and gestures 2° to language barrier.

Self-Care: Pt depend for bathing and dressing. She is able to perform min self-grooming tasks with the support of the w/c.

Equipment: Pt currently has no adaptive equipment.

C. **What are Schoci's goals?**

According to Korean tradition, when a family member becomes disabled the family is responsible for taking of him or her. The disabled family member is not expected to contribute to the care and maintenance of himself or herself or the household. Schoci and her family feel strongly that they must maintain this tradition in their household. Schoci will return home to her sister's family and be taken care of, regardless of the level of care she requires.

D. **How can Schoci reach her goals?**

1. Identify Schoci's strengths and weaknesses.

   Strengths

   ❑ supportive family with traditional views
   ❑ (L) UE functioning (generally)
   ❑ head and postural control

   Weaknesses

   ❑ orientation
   ❑ (R) UE status
   ❑ (L) UE strength
   ❑ transfer status
   ❑ sitting balance
   ❑ bed mobility
   ❑ perception
   ❑ self-care status
   ❑ communication

2. Identify the major skills Schoci or her family will need in order for Schoci to go home. (List long-term goals.)

   ❑ extensive home care techniques (Complete independence of skills not desired because of the traditional beliefs of the family.)
   ❑ safe transfer and bed mobility techniques
   ❑ increase Schoci's (L) UE strength and sitting balance to enhance the family's ability to care for Schoci.

3. What specific skills and equipment needs must be addressed for Schoci to work toward the major skills listed previously? Why? (List short-term goals.)

   a. Increase bed mobility to independent. Allow patient to perform weight-shifting in bed so family does not need to monitor her every 2 hours. Mobility also assists family members during care routines.
   b. Increase sitting balance for the patient's safety and to assist the family with general care.
   c. Increase (L) UE strength to enable Schoci to assist with her self-care without interfering with the family's traditional beliefs.

4. Identify two specific activities per area addressed in Section 3.

   ❏ Justify each activity in relation to Schoci's weaknesses.
   ❏ Explain how you would upgrade each activity.

   a. Increase bed mobility to independent. Allow patient to perform weight-shifting in bed so family does not need to monitor her every 2 hours. Mobility also assists family members during care routines.

   Activity One

   Justification

   Upgrade

   Activity Two

   Justification

   Upgrade

b. Increase sitting balance to help ensure the patient's safety and to assist the family with general care.

Activity One

Justification

Upgrade

Activity Two

Justification

Upgrade

c. Increase (L) UE strength to enable Schoci to assist with her self-care without interfering with the family's traditional beliefs.

Activity One

Justification

Upgrade

Activity Two

Justification

Upgrade

To complete the next questions, disregard the family's views on tradition by using the information in Question C in the place of the preceding information in Question C. Determine how this will change the treatment plan.

C. What are Schoci's goals?

Schoci and her family would like her to return home with her sister's family. She would like to contribute to the household care in some capacity and would like to be as independent as possible.

D. How can Schoci reach these goals?

1. Identify Schoci's strengths and weaknesses.

Strengths

- ❏ Schoci's desire to return to functional independence and her family's support
- ❏ (L) UE functioning (generally)
- ❏ head and postural control

Weaknesses

- ❏ orientation
- ❏ (R) UE status
- ❏ (L) UE strength
- ❏ transfer status
- ❏ sitting balance
- ❏ bed mobility
- ❏ perception
- ❏ self-care status
- ❏ communication

2. Identify the major skills Schoci and her family will need to enable Schoci to go home. (List long-term goals.)

- ❏ become oriented to her environment
- ❏ increase (R) UE functioning and/or learn to protect the arm
- ❏ increase transferring ability in order to be as indep as possible
- ❏ show good compensation for perception deficits to increase safety
- ❏ be able to perform ADLs as independently as possible
- ❏ have a safe mode of functional mobility
- ❏ know one-handed techniques for ADLs and ILS

3. What specific skills and equipment will be needed in order to work toward the major skills listed previously? Why? (List short-term goals.)

   a. She will need to improve her dynamic sitting balance strength to assist with transfers and general mobility.
   b. She will need to become aware of her right visual deficits and learn compensation techniques.
   c. She will need to be able to dress and bathe herself and perform hygiene and grooming needs as independently as possible.
   d. Teach one-handed techniques for household functioning.

4. Identify two specific activities per area addressed in Section 3.

- ❏ Justify each activity in relation to Schoci's weaknesses.
- ❏ Explain how you would upgrade each activity.

a. She will need to improve her dynamic sitting balance strength to assist with transfers and general mobility.

Activity One

Justification

Upgrade

Activity Two

Justification

Upgrade

b. She will need to become aware of her right visual deficits and learn compensation techniques.

Activity One

Justification

Upgrade

Activity Two

Justification

Upgrade

c. She will need to be able to dress and bathe herself and perform hygiene and grooming needs as independently as possible.

Activity One

Justification

Upgrade

Activity Two

Justification

Upgrade

d. Teach one-handed techniques for household functioning.

Activity One

Justification

Upgrade

Activity Two

Justification

Upgrade

Stella is a 48 y/o WF. It is currently June.

Referral reads

OT for ADLs

Medical Chart Information

❏ L CVA

❏ Meds

❏ DM

❏ Pt married with 3 children; 1 daughter lives at home and is currently in high school. Her husband words during the day for a construction company.

Occupational Therapy Evaluation Summary

S: Interview indicates that pt was independent with ADLs prior to incident. She is home alone during the day and does all the cooking and housework. Prior to incident, she used no adaptive equipment.

O: Sitting balance G+; pt is able to reach her feet and cross her legs s̄ losing her balance on a firm surface, but has difficulty with these tasks on a soft surface such as her bed.

Standing balance F+; pt is able to stand and take min. challenges ex. perform counter and tabletop activities. Tends to lose her balance when reaching above or below her waist.

(R) UE status: P+ at shoulder; P at elbow/wrist; trace finger movement; PROM is WFL; Pt shows no pain or edema in (R) UE c̄ PROM.

(L) UE strength: AROM is WFL; strength is normal throughout.

Cognitive status: Pt displays no significant language problems. Her memory and judgment are intact. She is able to follow directions appropriately. She is completely oriented but shows minimum deficits with sequencing ADL tasks.

ADL status: Pt requires moderate (A) donning/doffing her shirt 2° to ↓'d use of (R) UE and poor sequencing of task. She requires moderate (A) to don socks 2° to ↓'d use of (R) UE. Pt requires minimum (A) to transfer in and out of tub, using transfer tub bench. She requires minimum (A) for bathing. She requires minimum (A) to use WBQC during household mobility 2° to difficulty c̄ dynamic standing balance. Pt requires (A) to reach areas above or below waist during kitchen activities 2° to balance difficulties.

A: Pt's strengths include her general cognitive status and her (L) side functioning. Her limitations include her ADL status and (R) UE functioning. Pt shows good rehab potential.

P: ↑ UE dressing to min (A) in 1 week

↑ standing balance to good in 1 week

↑ (R) shoulder strength to fair– in 1 week

Instructions from OTR:

❏ focus on ADLs in general

❏ focus on weight-shifting on (R) LE standing at a table

❏ initiate gravity-eliminated activities and min WB activities to (R) shoulder

❏ write three activities for each goal and upgrade.

ACTIVITY	UPGRADE

❑ write progress note: Assume all goals are met and the following:
  ❑ sitting balance ↑'d to normal; able to reach floor, etc.
  ❑ pt states she feels stronger every day
  ❑ sequencing has ↑'d to good for daily tasks
  ❑ choose one new area on which to work.

Phillip is a 9 y/o M admitted to a rehabilitation unit. The average length of stay is 6 months. No significant medical hx prior to injury. Trach tube extubation s/p 2 weeks. Colostomy bag and catheter placed s/p 3 weeks. Frontal and occipital lobe contusion c̄ diffuse lesions.

Referral reads

❏ CHI
❏ begin eval for ADLs

Medical chart information

The facility in which you work is interdisciplinary. It is common practice to work with the physical therapist on gross-motor skills and the speech pathologist on communication skills. Each session is described, including the goals of the physical therapist and the speech pathologist.

Physical therapy and occupational therapy information

Phillip has been brought to the department on a stretcher. He was a total lift to transfer, and he is lying on the mat. His facial expression and increased body tone indicate that he is crying. He appears to be in pain all over when you try to move him. Phillip shows flaccid tone throughout his body, except minimum reflexive movement in his upper and lower extremities. He shows minimum head control while sitting edge-of-mat, by moving his head left and right, but he requires a head rest for support at all times. You and the physical therapist have agreed it is too early to attempt any lower-extremity weight-bearing activities at this time.

Physical therapy goals

❏ Pt will tolerate PROM to all extremities.
❏ Pt will tolerate sitting EOM with total support for 1 min.

Speech pathology and occupational therapy information

Phillip is in a reclining w/c. He is unable to speak or move his lips effectively to mouth words. He can use his eyes to look right and left and identify some pictures and words by eye gaze. He is able to control his eye blinks. Phillip attempts to blow out a match, but his lips are not in the correct position, and he has minimum breath support. He cries s̄ sound when he cannot do a task he is asked to do.

Speech therapy goals

❑ Pt able to perform oral-motor exercises with modeling and visual cues (use of mirror).
❑ Pt able to identify four needs by using a communication board and eye gazes with setup.

Occupational therapy goals

A. Formulate each OTR recommendation into goal format. Wear hand splints 2 hrs on/off. Able to sit in supported w/c for 1 hr at a time. Shows minimum head control c̄ head rest removed (15 secs).

B. What w/c equipment would you suggest to the OTR?

C. Devise 3 activities that take into consideration y/n responses, orientation, ↑ general head control, eye gaze, and general methods to ease Phillip's fear of the situation. (Make sure activities are age-appropriate.)

ACTIVITIES	UPGRADE POSSIBILITIES

D. How do you explain the situation to Phillip in order to enhance his cooperation c̄ the plan that has been outlined?

You will need to organize a cooking group for therapy (see Figure 2.3). There are three patients whom the staff agrees would be appropriate for the group. Not all the patients are yours, so you have checked with the other therapists and received the information that follows.

Cheryl:

49 y/o F, mother of 4, pt expressive aphasic, Dx (R) CVA

Focus of therapy

- ❏ ↑ standing tolerance (5 min+)
- ❏ one-handed activities
- ❏ ↑ pt verbal direction following
- ❏ ↑ pt (L) UE strength

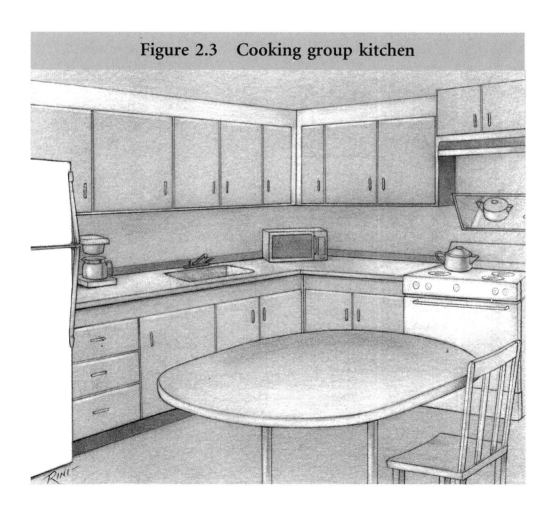

Figure 2.3   Cooking group kitchen

Warren:

68 y/o M, retired school teacher, Dx (R) BKA, has prosthesis, insulin-dependent DM

Focus of therapy

❏ ↑ household mobility c̄ cane
❏ ↑ weight shifting on (R) LE
❏ ↑ standing tolerance

Eleanor:

79 y/o F, homemaker, loves to work in the kitchen, Dx Parkinson's disease c̄ dementia

Focus of therapy

❏ following simple repetitive routines
❏ ↑ use of (B) UEs
❏ ↑ social involvement and orientation to surroundings

Planning the group

A. Before deciding on the menu, what do you need to consider for the safety of the patients?

B. Which discipline could you consult to assist with the menu and the food portions for each patient?

After consulting with the appropriate discipline, you and the patients have decided on this menu:

      roasted chicken breast (You have a simple menu card to follow.)
      fresh steamed carrots
      mashed potatoes (You plan to boil them before the actual meal time.)
      fresh fruit salad of apples, oranges, strawberries, and grapes

C. Assign tasks that would be appropriate for each of the patients according to the goals listed previously. Not all of the goals have to be addressed, and time is not a factor. Be sure to include tasks such as setting and clearing the table, cleaning up after the meal, and holding appropriately guided table conversations.

D. Formulate one goal for each patient related to the individual's listed deficits and the cooking activity.

You are assigned to an upper-extremity group that meets for 1 hour. There are currently three patients in the group, and they are not assigned to your caseload. The primary therapists gave you the following information about each patient. Assume any equipment or materials are available.

Nick:

62 y/o M, divorced, father of two grown sons, Dx (L) CVA

Focus of therapy

❏ practice lifting (L) UE to shoulder height and across his chest
❏ practice gross grasp (He has no isolated finger movement.)

Sara:

36 y/o F, mother of 1 young child, secretary, Dx (R) hand burn (no precautions)

Focus of therapy

❏ Practice fine-motor skills with (R) hand (She has isolated finger movement but needs to ↑ ROM in fingers and wrist.)

David:

28 y/o M, construction worker, Dx broken humerus, radius at the (R) elbow (no current precautions). Cast removal 3 days ago.

Focus of therapy

❏ Elbow is frozen at 75°; goal is to stretch out elbow with functional activities.

Planning the group

A. Choose an activity in which all three patients can participate and that can be completed in 1 hour. (Keep in mind the activity needs to be functional and age-appropriate.)

B. Assign tasks that would be appropriate for each of the patients according to the guidelines provided by the primary therapists.

C. Formulate one goal for each patient related to the individual's deficits and the activity you have chosen.

EXERCISE 2:10 Nursing Home Group

You are working in a nursing home with long-term-care patients. You have a group of patients you are seeing for 1 hour. Next week is Valentine's Day. Each patient has the following therapy focus. Assume any materials or equipment is available.

Earl:

89 y/o M, married, lives with wife in nursing home, HOH, no specific diagnosis

Focus of therapy

❑ Dynamic standing balance (Earl is able to walk s̄ an assistive device but tends to lose his balance when reaching high and low surfaces.)
❑ ↑ general orientation and sequencing skills

Martha:

78 y/o F, severe RA, widowed, has 2 daughters and 4 grandchildren who live out of state

Focus of therapy

❑ Martha's hands/fingers are not functional. ↑ gross movement and function with hands. Do not emphasize moving fingers but on using hands s̄ fingers. (You can use adaptive equipment as an option.)

Viola:

87 y/o F, widowed, Dx dementia and (L) CVA. Viola can follow simple directions and complete simple repetitive tasks with verbal cues.

Focus of therapy

❑ ↑ use of one-handed activities using (L) UE
❑ ↑ sitting balance; goal to ↑ pt's ability to reach items across the table height from w/c

Planning the group

A. Choose a functional activity related to Valentine's Day that all pts can participate in and that addresses each pt's goal. Task should be completed within 1 hour.

B. Assign tasks that would be appropriate for each of the pts according to the guidelines provided.

C. Formulate one goal for each pt related to the individual's deficits and the activity you have chosen.

You are working in a rehabilitation facility. You are assigned to a work activity group. The goal of the group is to prepare patients for vocational tasks. The group has been given a task from the Red Cross. The task is a mailing, described below next.

❑ Each envelope needs to have two pages stapled together and a brochure.
❑ Labels need to be put on the envelopes.
❑ Envelopes need to be sorted by zip code.
❑ There are 500 labels.
❑ The supplies will be delivered to the front desk downstairs in boxes and need to be returned to the front desk when the task is completed.

The patients in the group and their focus of therapy are listed next.

Eric:

27 y/o M, single, Dx of CHI 2° to MVA. Eric has full functional use of his UEs and LEs. His deficits relate to his cognitive status only.

Focus of therapy

❑ ↑ pt's ability to attend to a repetitive task for 10 minutes
❑ ↑ pt's ability to sequence tasks
❑ ↑ pt's orientation to place and topographical orientation

Larry:

34 y/o M, Dx paraplegia 2° to a diving accident. Larry has full UE functioning and no cognitive deficits.

Focus of therapy

❑ ↑ sitting balance to being able to reach the floor and overhead
❑ ↑ w/c mobility and ability to move items from one surface to another

Dorothy:

39 y/o F, Dx (R) CVA. She has no functional use of her (L) UE and requires min (A) to stand for 5 minutes at the table.

Focus of therapy

❑ ↑ high level cognitive ability (Example: complex sequencing.)
❑ ↑ standing tolerance at the table
❑ ↑ one-handed task abilities

A. Assign tasks that would be appropriate for each of the patients according to the guidelines provided.

B. Formulate one goal for each pt related to the individual's deficits and the activity provided.

**TREATMENT
PLANNING
PROCESS**

Mark is sitting on the edge of the mat working with a set of pegs at a table. The pegs are 1 inch in diameter, and they are different colors. They fit in a board with precarved holes. He is taking the pegs out of a bucket and placing them on the board. Based on the information provided in the next sections, describe how you would alter this task to challenge each deficit listed by answering the following questions. Other pieces of therapeutic equipment can be added to the tasks (see Figure 2.4).

Part 1

Mark is working on sitting balance. He is able to sit comfortably on the edge of the mat and do this activity.

A. How would you upgrade the activity?

B. Formulate one goal related to the upgraded task.

**Figure 2.4
Mark**

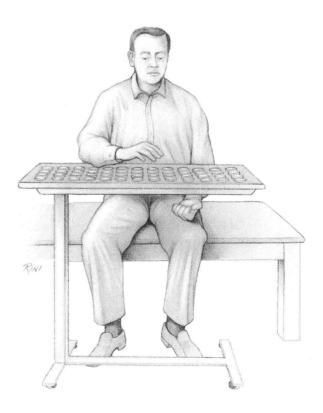

Part 2

Mark is working on strengthening his left upper extremity. His arm can comfortably perform this activity.

A. How would you upgrade this activity?

B. Formulate one goal related to the upgraded task.

Part 3

Mark is confused and unable to sequence simple tasks. He is able to follow directions for the activity listed previously by just picking and placing random pegs.

A. How would you upgrade this activity?

B. Formulate one goal related to the upgraded task.

EXERCISE 2:13 Mabel

Mabel is 68 y/o. She has a diagnosis of hip fracture, and she has a medical history of dementia. Mabel has been living with her daughter and son-in-law for the past 3 years. During her initial OT evaluation, you ask Mabel to raise her arms. She is not able to raise them. Then you give her a towel and ask her to fold it. She folds it perfectly, including shaking it out. You ask her to stand up. She tries but is unable to coordinate the movements to stand. You ask her to get some butter out of the refrigerator. She stands up but requires minimum assistance to walk to the refrigerator. Mabel is not able to follow directions, but she can perform spontaneous functional activities. She has no medical restrictions, and yet shows discomfort when bending to touch her feet.

A. The therapist did not include a goal to follow directions or for using adaptive equipment. Why?

B. Assuming you have an apartment setup and any equipment you need, list three activities for each goal listed next.

❏ Pt able to perform functional transfers for everyday living independently.

   1.

   2.

   3.

❏ Pt able to stand with minimum challenges and equal weight-bearing on LEs for 10 minutes. (Assume minimum challenge is moving arms between shoulder and waist height.)

   1.

   2.

   3.

❏ Pt able to don/doff shoes and socks c̄ SBA. (Analyze the movements needed for this activity in relation to the injury.)

   1.

   2.

   3.

C. Assume that Mabel has met all the previous goals. Write three goals to work on for next week.

   1.

   2.

   3.

EXERCISE 2:14 Peter

Peter is a 73 y/o BM c̄ a Dx of CVA. April is his occupational therapy assistant. She has been working c̄ Peter for 2 wks. She is at her desk talking to Sally, another occupational therapy assistant. April tells Sally she does not know what is wrong with Peter.

"He has a lot of potential for recovery, but he will not work on his arm or do any of the perception activities I give him. I try to make his activities interesting. His arm and perception are the only things I am focusing on right now. I guess he is just not motivated to get better," she says.

April is off the next day, and Sally fills in for her and sees Peter. Below are descriptions of the therapy sessions with Peter and each of the therapists.

April and Peter

April: "Good morning, Peter; let's work on your arm first today. I thought we would practice bowling, because you used to be on a league." (She brings out a small plastic ball and sets up the plastic pins.) April has to physically help Peter with all the movement for the activity.

Peter: "I am tired; can we stop?"

April: "Okay, we will rest for a couple of minutes. Then I have a peg design for you to work on."

Peter: "Great!"

Sally and Peter

Sally: "Good morning, Peter. My name is Sally. April is not here today, so I will be working with you. I see from your treatment plan you are working on your right arm and perception skills. What would you like to do this morning?"

Peter: "I want to work on my walking. What is 'perception' anyway?"

Sally: "Perception is the ability to understand exactly what you see. For example, if we are both going to walk up a flight of stairs, I may think the steps are 4 inches high and you may think they are 6 inches high. We both see the steps, but one of us is going to have problems when we try to lift our feet to go up. Now you want to work on walking. Okay. Let's start with standing at the table. You should be able to stand before you can walk." (Sally helps Peter stand at the table using both arms to push up from the w/c.)

Sally: "You stand pretty well. Now let's challenge your balance a little. Pick up these pegs and put them in this basket, first with your left hand, then with your right hand. You should feel your weight shifting from hip to hip just like walking. (Peter stands about 10 minutes and uses his left and right hands for the activity. He requires minimum assistance for use of his right hand.)

Sally: "Are you getting tired?" (She feels Peter's hips and knees weakening.)

Peter: "No, I'm fine."

Sally: "Well, I'm getting tired, so let's sit down." (She helps him sit back in the w/c using both of his hands to lower himself.) "Now, Peter, remember what I told you about perception and the steps?"

Peter: "Yes, I understand now."

Sally: "Okay. I would like you to copy this block design to work on your ability to trust what you see."

Peter: "Sure." (Peter finishes the design. Sally assists him with a few corrections.)

Peter: "I guess I do have a problem with that. Thanks, Sally, and I'll see you this afternoon."

Based on the treatment session answer the following questions:

A. Did both April and Sally work on the same goals for Peter?

B. Were the activities developed by April inappropriate for his skill level?

C. Why did Sally get such a different response from Peter?

D. Does Peter have a motivation problem? If not, why was April having such a difficult time with Peter?

E. If you were Sally, would you say anything to April? If so, what would you say?

F. Does a patient have the right not to work on a specific area of dysfunction, even if he or she had good potential for recovery?

Bob is a 58 y/o M who suffered a CVA 5 days ago. He is a large man. His hobbies include fishing, hunting, and working on cars. He was employed as a foreman at a car factory. Bob was very active; his wife says he was never home because he always found something to do. Bob is expressively and receptively aphasic. He has fair–strength on the right side of his body. He has come to the department for the first time in a wheelchair. You introduce yourself. Bob cries very hard and points to his mouth and hand.

A. What do you say or do? How would you explain to him what happened and why he is here to see you? (Remember, he is aphasic, so any explanations need to use one- to two-word phrases and gestures.)

B. The OTR has chosen goal areas of increasing wheelchair mobility to gain immediate independence and is working on sitting balance. Why would she want to work on both immediate independence and functional recovery through development process at the same time?

Eleanor is a 79 y/o F who suffered a CVA 7 days ago. She is brought to the department in a wheelchair. Her head is positioned severely to the right. You begin your initial interview c̄ her, and she suddenly stops and leans very close to you. She says, "I think I am losing my mind." A tear slides down her cheek. She continues, "I am hearing voices." With further questioning, you find out that when people talk to her on her left side or the left side of the room, she does not turn her head. Her hospital bed is by the window, and she is not aware that she has a roommate in the bed to her left. The OTR has indicated in her evaluation that Eleanor has severe visual neglect.

A. How do you explain this situation to her? (Remember to explain it to her in terms she can understand.)

B. Is there anything you can suggest that will make her more comfortable in her room?

Dr. Bones has been referred to the OT Department after a THR. He has been retired for about 3 years.

Dr. Bones: What am I doing here?

You reply:

Alan is 48 y/o. He has had a BKA of the left lower extremity and has received his prosthesis. He is a stockbroker and, during the initial interview, appeared eager to get back to work. He has told you about a pain he has been feeling in his left foot and leg. He says, "I know that is ridiculous because my leg is gone, but it really hurts."

A. How would you explain phantom pain to Alan? (Review definition of phantom pain.)

B. Alan also asks, "Why do I need to waste my time here anyway?" What do you say to him?

Gerry is 27 y/o. He is mentally retarded and has lived at home all of his life. He is functioning at a 5-year-old developmental level. Gerry had an MI 4 days ago. He enjoys rap music and coloring.

Therapy Plan

1. The patient will tolerate 10 minutes of tabletop activities in 1 week.

2. The patient will perform upper-extremity dressing with minimum assistance in 1 week. (Watch precautions of hand-over-hand.)

3. The patient will tolerate 5 minutes of standing actively using hands with counter support in 1 week.

A. Gerry looks scared and asks, "Where is my mommy?" What would you tell him?

B. Choose three activities per goal and upgrade option.

The patient will tolerate 10 minutes of tabletop activities in 1 week.

ACTIVITY	UPGRADE

The patient will perform upper-extremity dressing with minimum assistance in 1 week. (Watch precautions of hand-over-hand.)

ACTIVITY	UPGRADE

The patient will tolerate 5 minutes of standing actively using hands with counter support in 1 week.

ACTIVITY	UPGRADE

C. Gerry asks, "Why am I here? What are we going to do?" How would you explain the situation to him?

Joe is a 27 y/o M. His diagnosis is multiple gunshot wounds c̄ incomplete T5-6. Joe is 6'2" and 230#. As you approach the nursing station and pull the chart, the nurse says, "That man is wild; he yells and curses at everyone. He has been cussing the doctors and nurses out for the last 3 days. Good luck." The social hx indicates he is a high school dropout and has been working on a loading dock for 8 months and has a girlfriend. The medical chart indicates a hx of drug and alcohol abuse.

A. Knowing Joe's hx and his current situation, what are the possible causes for his behavior?

B. As you enter the room, he is lying in bed staring out the window. How do you introduce yourself and how do you explain OT?

EXERCISE 2:21 Jessica

Jessica is a 10 y/o girl with a diagnosis of CHI as a result of a motor vehicle accident. She has been in a rehabilitation unit for 4 months. She is currently able to use her right hand to operate a joystick on computer games without difficulty; however, she is not able to use grasp or release or hold a pencil. She remains very flaccid throughout her body and may have the potential to walk, but only with years of continued therapy. Her cognitive functioning is WFL for her age.

About a month ago, you and the occupational therapist felt that she could successfully benefit from an electric wheelchair. Jessica also saw a patient with an electric wheelchair and has been asking what she has to be able to do to have a chair like that. The occupational therapist discussed this with her father and mother. The father was very angry with the idea, and her mother was very quiet.

The next day, Jessica and her father came down to therapy, and Jessica said, "I don't want an electric wheelchair; I will be walking soon." The entire rehabilitation team feels that Jessica can begin school in August with the right equipment.

A. Why did Jessica's father become angry?

B. The father became angry and very verbal during a treatment session. What do you do or say?

C. Based on the assumption that Jessica's right arm movement is the only controllable movement she has, what other equipment ideas could you suggest for going back to school?

References

Day, D. J. (1973). A systems diagram for teaching treatment planning. *American Journal of Occupational Therapy, 27,* 239–243.

DiMatteo, M. R. (1991). *The psychology of health, illness, and medical care: An individual perspective.* Pacific Grove, CA: Brooks/Cole.

DiMatteo, M. R., & DiNicola, D. D. (1982). *Achieving patient compliance: The psychology of the medical practitioner's role.* New York: Pergamon Press.

Hammond, D. C., Hepworth, D. H., & Smith, V. G. (1977). *Improving therapeutic communication.* San Francisco, CA: Jossey-Bass.

Hemphill, B. J. (1982). The evaluative process. In B. J. Hemphill (Ed)., *Psychiatric occupational therapy* (pp. 3–12). Thorofare, NJ: Slack.

Kuntavanish, A. A. (1987). *Occupational therapy documentation.* Bethesda, MD: American Occupational Therapy Association.

Lau, R. R., & Hartman, K. A. (1983). Common-sense representations of common illnesses. *Health Psychology, 2,* 167–185.

Mandler, G., & Kahn, M. (1960). Discrimination of changes in heart rate: Two unsuccessful attempts. *Journal of the Experimental Analysis of Behavior, 3,* 21–25.

McKinlay, J. B. (1972). Some approaches and problems in the study of the use of services: An overview. *Journal of Health and Social Behavior, 13,* 115–152.

Nerenz, D. R., & Leventhal, H. (1983). Self-regulation theory in chronic illness. In T. G. Burish & L. A. Bradley (Eds.), *Coping with chronic disease: Research and applications* (pp. 13–38). New York: Academic Press.

Pedretti, L. W. (1985). Treatment planning. In L. W. Pedretti (Ed.), *Occupational therapy* (2nd ed., pp. 22–29). Princeton, NJ: Mosely.

Ryan, S. E. (1993). *The certified occupational therapy assistant.* Thorofare, NJ: Slack.

CHAPTER 3

Discharge Process and Home Care

Objectives

After completing the exercises in this chapter, the student should be able to:

❏ identify discharge settings and compare the levels of services offered at each setting

❏ provide continued therapy recommendations according to an individual's discharge placement

❏ identify characteristics of home-program development

❏ develop home programs for patients based on their physical and cognitive limitations and rehabilitation needs.

Introduction

Nancy is an occupational therapy assistant student completing her final affiliation. She has been working with Joe for 2 weeks. Joe suffered a subdural hematoma and was making good progress in regaining his independence.

When Nancy first started seeing Joe, there was no indication of how long he would be hospitalized. Nancy was positive about their working relationship and the treatment plan. During weekly team meetings with the OTR to review Joe's total treatment plan, she was informed that Joe would be discharged home by the end of the month, which was in 2 weeks.

After the meeting, Nancy and the OTR reviewed Joe's treatment plan with the new discharge information to make adjustments. As they reviewed the treatment options that would allow her to meet the time restraints, she began to feel that this discharge plan was very unfair to Joe in terms of his rehabilitation process. Every treatment option they examined made her feel like she was putting a bandage on Joe's deficits rather than progressing him to his fullest potential of recovery. Nancy feared that once Joe was discharged from the facility, his rehabilitation would stop, and he would lose his current level of functioning.

Therapists are taught to see the potential of individuals during the therapeutic process—in fact, their education focuses entirely on seeing a patient's potential for independence at all levels of functioning. Nancy and her supervising occupational therapist found Joe's potential and had been working with him to recover his independence. However, many external factors influence the recovery process.

A number of these factors have been reviewed in the first two chapters of this workbook. Because of these factors, a therapist may often feel that a patient is not receiving the full benefit of therapeutic recovery. Many times the therapist believes that if patients do not receive treatment from the therapist's clinic, they will have no chance of recovery.

Section I   Health Care Continuum

The entire health care services environment has a great deal of influence on a person's rehabilitation and recovery process. Access to and use of health care services are changing constantly. Today's health care environment is particularly dynamic because of the nationwide focus on reducing health care cost.

Health care should be viewed as a continuum of services that provides support to individuals for recovery from an illness or for readapting to the community and life roles. The occupational therapy services delivery model designed by Carolyn Baum (Christiansen & Baum, 1991) provides a description of the levels of occupational therapy services that are commonly provided in today's health care environment. Figure 3.1 expands on the average service definitions for the occupational therapy services. Understanding the basic services that are provided, funding and

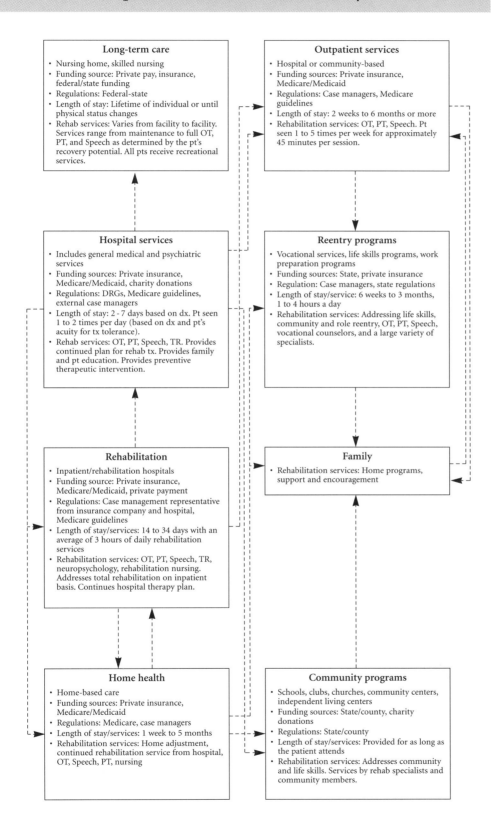

Long-term care
- Nursing home, skilled nursing
- Funding source: Private pay, insurance, federal/state funding
- Regulations: Federal-state
- Length of stay: Lifetime of individual or until physical status changes
- Rehab services: Varies from facility to facility. Services range from maintenance to full OT, PT, and Speech as determined by the pt's recovery potential. All pts receive recreational services.

Outpatient services
- Hospital or community-based
- Funding sources: Private insurance, Medicare/Medicaid
- Regulations: Case managers, Medicare guidelines
- Length of stay: 2 weeks to 6 months or more
- Rehabilitation services: OT, PT, Speech. Pt seen 1 to 5 times per week for approximately 45 minutes per session.

Hospital services
- Includes general medical and psychiatric services
- Funding sources: Private insurance, Medicare/Medicaid, charity donations
- Regulations: DRGs, Medicare guidelines, external case managers
- Length of stay: 2 - 7 days based on dx. Pt seen 1 to 2 times per day (based on dx and pt's acuity for tx tolerance).
- Rehab services: OT, PT, Speech, TR. Provides continued plan for rehab tx. Provides family and pt education. Provides preventive therapeutic intervention.

Reentry programs
- Vocational services, life skills programs, work preparation programs
- Funding sources: State, private insurance
- Regulation: Case managers, state regulations
- Length of stay/service: 6 weeks to 3 months, 1 to 4 hours a day
- Rehabilitation services: Addressing life skills, community and role reentry, OT, PT, Speech, vocational counselors, and a large variety of specialists.

Rehabilitation
- Inpatient/rehabilitation hospitals
- Funding source: Private insurance, Medicare/Medicaid, private payment
- Regulations: Case management representative from insurance company and hospital, Medicare guidelines
- Length of stay/services: 14 to 34 days with an average of 3 hours of daily rehabilitation services
- Rehabilitation services: OT, PT, Speech, TR, neuropsychology, rehabilitation nursing. Addresses total rehabilitation on inpatient basis. Continues hospital therapy plan.

Family
- Rehabilitation services: Home programs, support and encouragement

Home health
- Home-based care
- Funding sources: Private insurance, Medicare/Medicaid
- Regulations: Medicare, case managers
- Length of stay/services: 1 week to 5 months
- Rehabilitation services: Home adjustment, continued rehabilitation service from hospital, OT, Speech, PT, nursing

Community programs
- Schools, clubs, churches, community centers, independent living centers
- Funding sources: State/county, charity donations
- Regulations: State/county
- Length of stay/services: Provided for as long as the patient attends
- Rehabilitation services: Addresses community and life skills. Services by rehab specialists and community members.

Adapted with permission from Baum, C. & Christiansen, C. (1991). *Occupational therapy: Overcoming human performance deficits.* Thorofare, NJ: Slack.

regulation issues, and average length of rehabilitation services in health care programs can help the therapist be part of the health care continuum and provide effective discharge recommendations for patients. These descriptions are not completely accurate because of the changing nature of health care and the complexity of the system.

As illustrated in the figure, an individual generally enters the health care system through the hospital or other medical services. The patient then can continue to a rehabilitation facility or long-term care or can return to home with supportive therapy.

Patients who return home can receive services through outpatient therapy, home health, reentry, or community programs. Patients who return home also often receive an informal type of therapy treatment by their families. A well-educated family and support systems can continue to improve the patient's level of independence.

Hospital Services

Hospital services include a large variety of medically based treatments. Most physical and psychiatric services begin in a hospital setting. Although many hospitals are considered nonprofit organizations, they still need to consider financial reimbursement in order to maintain staff and equipment. The common funding sources are private insurance, federal and state funding (i.e., Medicare and Medicaid), donations, and private payment by consumers.

Regulators that affect a patient's length of stay and the services that will be provided are the diagnosis related groups (DRGs), state and federal guidelines (i.e., Medicare and Medicaid), and case managers who represent private insurance companies.

Today the average length of the hospital stay ranges from 2 to 7 days, depending on the diagnosis. The common rehabilitation services provided are occupational therapy, physical therapy, speech, and therapeutic recreation. Patients are seen 1 or 2 times per day, depending on the patient's diagnosis and endurance. The primary focus of occupational therapy treatment is therapeutic intervention, preventative treatment techniques, family education, and provision of a therapeutic plan to assist with discharge recommendations.

Long-Term Care

Long-term care includes nursing homes and skilled nursing facilities. The term *long-term care* is used frequently because of the stigma associated with nursing homes. They are frequently identified as a place to wait to die, regardless of the services provided.

There is a new trend developing in the long-term-care institution. Many facilities are providing rehabilitation services that focus on independent living skills within the facility. This method is intended to decrease the burden of care or facilitate the patient's transition back to his or her family and home.

The changes in long-term care evolved from the economic need to decrease the cost of care to the patient. It is important to know in advance whether rehabilitation services will be available to patients being placed in long-term care facilities in order to be able to adjust the treatment recommendations according to the patient's needs.

The funding sources for long-term care generally are the federal and state governments, insurance companies, and private payments. Regulations are instituted along state and federal guidelines. The length of stay can range from the lifetime of the individual to until there has been a physical or mental status change that may indicate a potential for functional independence. The primary rehabilitation service provided is physical therapy; occupational therapy, speech, and therapeutic recreation are also provided by physician referral.

Traditionally, the focus of long-term-care therapeutic intervention is maintenance and recreational programming. A consulting occupational therapist may provide services for 30 to 60 patients. Basic maintenance activities, such as passive range of motion (PROM) and bed positioning, are generally done by the nursing staff after a consultation with physical therapy or occupational therapy.

Rehabilitation Services

A rehabilitation unit or hospital is designed to provide intensive rehabilitation services once the patient is medically stable. Rehabilitation services are provided by occupational therapy, physical therapy, speech, therapeutic recreation, and nursing. The average length of stay is 7 to 34 days, and most facilities offer at least 3 hours of direct therapy care per day.

Funding sources generally are private insurance, Medicare, and private payments. The rehabilitation process is regulated by federal guidelines and case managers representing private insurance companies. The focus of therapy is to provide an intense, total rehabilitation program that is also a continuation of the therapy process initiated in the acute care facility.

Outpatient Services

The current trend for rehabilitation care is to improve and expand outpatient services. This is viewed as a cost-effective method of delivering health care services. The patient receives the benefit of rehabilitation care in a hospital or clinical setting while at home, so the facilities do not incur the expense of 24-hour patient care.

Traditionally, most outpatient care was delivered through the hospital. Today, many different types of facilities specialize in outpatient therapy. Hospitals have developed satellite facilities, physicians' offices provide therapy, and a growing number of clinics are operated by therapists. Funding sources generally are private payment, private insurance, and Medicare. The current trend is for the system to be regulated by federal and state case managers.

The length of service varies greatly. A patient may be seen 1 to 5 times a week; the diagnosis and patient's status determine the duration of treatment.

Rehabilitation services also vary with the type of clinic: physical therapy, occupational therapy, and speech are the major disciplines involved with outpatient rehabilitation. For example, staffing for an outpatient hand clinic usually includes occupational therapists and physical therapists. Outpatient services for neurological disorders includes occupational therapy, physical therapy, and speech.

Home Health Care

Many individuals receive home health services. A therapist will go to the person's home and provide treatment. The funding sources are private payment, private insurance, and Medicare. The system is regulated by Medicare guidelines and case managers. The length of service also varies, depending on the patient's need, usually ranging from 1 week to 3 months.

The patient typically is seen 1 to 3 times per week. The primary focus of home health services is to assist with the patient's adjustment to functioning in the home. Services are provided by physical therapy, occupational therapy, speech therapy, and nursing. Frequently, the patient must be home-bound to receive these services.

Reentry Programs

Reentry programs are designed to provide therapeutic intervention for life skills and for community and life-role reentry. The focus of these programs is return to work programs, transitional living, driver retraining and adaptation, technology center, head injury program, and vocational services. The programs are funded by state governments and private insurance. Regulation is provided by the state and case managers. The length of service is 6 weeks to 3 months. The programs provide service for 1 to 4 hours a day with each patient. The programs provide a large variety of disciplines, including occupational therapy, physical therapy, speech therapy, neuropsychology, vocational counseling, and therapeutic recreation.

Community Programs

Many community-based programs provide various degrees of rehabilitation care. Schools, clubs, churches, community centers, and independent living centers provide a range of therapeutic and support services for individuals who need assistance. The funding sources for some of these programs are the state and county governments, as well as charitable donations. Regulations are instituted by the state and county. The patients can participate in programs for as long as they are qualified to attend.

The staff includes some rehabilitation specialists, such as occupational therapists or physical therapists, but these programs also are supervised by members of the community. Many of these community programs provide family support and education. They also can be used as respite care resources.

The discharge summary is the responsibility of the OTR, although the COTA can contribute in great length to the process. When the goals set by the OTR and COTA are met, and OT services are no longer indicated, it is the responsibility of the COTA to inform the OTR. In some cases, the goals cannot be met for some reason, and again the OTR needs to be consulted. The COTA may not independently discharge a patient without input from the OTR.

In most situations, the occupational therapist is not responsible for making the entire discharge placement decision. Frequently, the occupational therapist has no control over these issues but can provide valuable recommendations that influence the discharge placement process. When discharge placement arrangements are determined, it is the therapist's responsibility to assist the patient with the transition by making recommendations and education to the patient, family members, and future facility.

For example, Thelma is an 84 y/o woman who suffered a stroke. She will be placed in a long-term-care facility. The occupational therapist providing her care in the current facility may make the following recommendations:

To future facility:

- ❏ OT p.r.n. to monitor splint wearing schedule, w/c & bed positioning
- ❏ Splint wearing schedule: 2 hrs on/2 hrs off

To patient:

- ❏ Provide information to Thelma about therapeutic activities that will be available to ease her transition.

To family:

- ❏ Provide family education related to PROM and benefits of bed positioning and getting out of bed as Thelma tolerates. This will enable the family members to be able to participate in her care if they desire, and they will be informed advocates for Thelma as well.

Practical Application

Complete exercises 3:1–3:6. Review the information provided and determine an appropriate occupational therapy recommendation of continued therapy services.

Section II   Home Program Development

A well-developed home program is a controlled educational mechanism for patients and caregivers to continue a therapeutic treatment plan independently. It also can serve as a plan for a safe transition to encourage a patient to be reintroduced to life roles in the home and community.

Frequently, after a hospitalization or the rehabilitative process, the patient and family members are unclear about what the patient can do safely on returning home. A home program should address concerns of the patient and family members to ease this transition.

Home programs also provide intervention strategies that enhance therapeutic and medical recovery. For example, suppose a woman had a surgical procedure to replace the metacarpal (MC) joints in her hand. The initial home program provided by the occupational therapist would include an exercise plan and strategies to reduce scarring and edema.

Components of a home program should include an explanation of the purpose and goals of the exercises or recommendations, as well as written instructions that consider the patient's level of understanding. The therapist also should provide the patient with his or her name and business telephone number in case the patient has any questions once the program at home has been implemented.

An explanation of the purpose and goals of the home program should be reviewed with the patient and the primary caregiver. The explanation should be reviewed verbally, and the patient or caregiver should be allowed time during the occupational therapy session to practice the recommendations and ask questions. A brief explanation should be included in the written directions to enable the patients or caregivers to review it when they get home.

This process may appear redundant; however, DiMatteo (1991) has indicated that there are many factors that interfere with the patient's ability to completely understand treatment recommendations. For example, many times health professionals communicate information in medical jargon or in terms that are unfamiliar to the patient. Other times, the patient's anxiety level may be so high during the therapeutic process that it can interfere with memorization and learning.

Sometimes people are reluctant to ask questions when they are provided with new information. They do not want to appear as if they are not intelligent enough to understand the process that is being explained.

Finally, the person's actual level of intelligence and the ability to relate to a new disability can affect the learning process. Providing a clear explanation, an opportunity to practice, and a brief written explanation can be effective in overcoming these communication barriers and will help ensure that the individual will follow through with the plan.

Providing written directions can be difficult, especially for those patients who have impaired reading ability. Pictures and diagrams may be the patient's only way of following the program. However, patients with perception deficits may find it difficult to follow diagrams. Therefore, providing an understandable home program may be as challenging to a therapist's creative ability as preparing the treatment plan itself.

The therapist should always provide his or her name, business telephone, and credentials with every home program. A patient may feel more comfortable calling the therapist than the physician if he or she is having complications or symptom

The Home Program

❑ Explanation of the purpose and goals of the exercises

❑ Written instructions

❑ Therapist's name and business phone number

changes. Also, patients or primary caregivers may have questions related to the program once they are at home. (See Figure 3.2.)

The therapists often provide three major types of information in home programs: energy conservation or protection, exercises, and suggestions for reintegrating the patient into his or her family role or activities. A program may include only one type of information or may have all three types, depending on the diagnosis and the amount of information the therapist has available.

For instance, a therapist who works with orthopedic patients may provide a home program for a patient with a total hip replacement after seeing him or her 1 day. The home program will be different for a patient with a total hip replacement who has been seen for 1 week. There will be similarities in preparation and exercises; however, the therapist who has seen the patient for 1 week will be able to provide more complete information in relation to life role reintegration.

Practical Application

Complete exercises 3:1–3:10. Provide written home recommendations for each patient.

Read each patient description carefully. Answer the following questions as if you were going to make recommendations to your supervisor.

Clifford is 68 y/o. He suffered a (R) CVA. He is a retired airplane pilot. Clifford is married and has two grown daughters who live in the same town. He enjoys golfing and spending time with his family. Clifford also enjoys visiting in his neighborhood.

Phase of Rehabilitation

Clifford is in a hospital rehabilitation unit. He has been receiving 3 hours of intensive rehab services a day for the past 5 weeks.

Living Situation

Clifford lives c̄ his wife in a one-floor, two-bedroom home. His wife has no significant physical or cognitive limitations. Clifford spends a great deal of time visiting his friends in the neighborhood.

Current Status

Clifford is ambulating short distances c̄ a small-base quad cane. His (L) UE has shown progressive recovery, from being flaccid to Clifford's being able to use it as a gross (A). He requires min-to-SBA for bathing and dressing c̄ the use of a transfer tub bench. Clifford has no significant cognitive deficits. His memory, judgment, and safety skills are intact.

Reimbursement Options

❑ home health care
❑ continued rehabilitation inpatient care
❑ outpatient services
❑ long-term care

A. In your opinion, would Clifford benefit from further occupational therapy rehabilitation services?

B. What level of care would you recommend?

C. Provide an outline for a therapy plan you would recommend for the next level of rehabilitative services that you choose.

D. Would you recommend any type of community programs for Clifford and his family?

EXERCISE 3:2 Bill

Bill is 53 y/o. He had an aneurysm that burst 2 weeks ago. Bill is married c̄ 2 sons and a daughter. He enjoys fishing and bowling. Bill works in construction. Both he and his wife are very active in their church community.

Phase of Rehabilitation

Bill is in an acute care hospital. He has just become medically stable and is being transferred out of the ICU. He has received OT and PT services.

Living Situation

Bill lives c̄ his wife in a second-floor apartment. His wife is a petite woman c̄ mild arthritis in her hands. Bill managed all the household finances.

Current Status

Bill has been medically stable for 2 days. He is alert for about ½ hour at a time but is disoriented and confused. He is beginning to tolerate sitting up on the side of the bed and showing some isolated finger movement in his affected UE. Bill can tolerate doing exercises supine for about 15 min c̄ his unaffected UE and LE. The OT and PT working with Bill have decided to begin getting him up in a w/c.

Reimbursement Options

❏ home health care
❏ inpatient rehabilitation
❏ long-term care

A. In your opinion, would Bill benefit from further occupational therapy rehabilitative services?

B. What level of care would you recommend?

C. Provide an outline for a therapy plan that you would recommend for the next level of rehabilitative services you choose.

D. Would you recommend any type of community programs to the patient and his family?

Valerie is 36 y/o. She was hit by a car 10 days ago. She suffered fractures of the (R) femur and (R) radius and has a crushed (R) wrist. She is a wife and mother of two children, Sarah who is 8 y/o and Nick who is 10 y/o. Valerie enjoys being a home-maker. She also enjoys sewing and needlework.

Phase of Recovery

Valerie has been in a rehabilitation center for 1 week. She has been receiving OT and PT services 2 x a day.

Living Situation

Valerie lives c̄ her family. Her sister lives a block away and has been caring for Valerie's children while she has been in the hospital. Valerie's sister is prepared to help her with the transition to home. Valerie's home has two levels and a basement. The bedrooms and bathroom are on the second floor, and the laundry facilities are in the basement.

Current Status

Valerie's femur is healing well. She is ambulating without an assistive device, but she still has difficulty manipulating the stairs because of a walking cast. Valerie has had two surgeries on her wrist since the accident. Her wrist cast has been removed, and the physician has ordered AROM as the pt tolerates. Valerie is indep c̄ bathing, dressing, and most other ADL skills, using adaptive techniques learned in OT.

Reimbursement Options

❏ home health care
❏ outpatient services
❏ reentry programs

A. In your opinion, would Valerie benefit from further occupational therapy rehabilitative services?

B. What level of care would you recommend?

C. Provide an outline for a therapy plan that you would recommend for the next level of rehabilitative services that you choose.

D. Would you recommend any type of community programs to the patient and her family?

EXERCISE 3:4 Imogene

Imogene is 83 y/o. Two weeks ago, she fell in her home and broke her hip. She underwent a THR surgical procedure. Imogene has four children who have their own families and live out of town. She is a retired housewife, and her husband passed away 8 years ago. When Imogene was asked about her interests, she said she kept busy. However, she was not able to identify any of her specific interests or hobbies.

Phase of Recovery

Imogene is receiving rehab services in a skilled nursing facility. She is being seen by a PT and OT.

Living Situation

Imogene lives alone in her two-story home. Her children keep in touch c̄ her by telephone, and two of her daughters visit about 1 week a year. One daughter said that every visit her mom gets older, but she is still managing to take care of herself. The social worker contacted one of Imogene's neighbors. The neighbor indicated that Imogene has been keeping to herself the past couple of years and that she has been checking on Imogene regularly. The social worker indicated that Imogene's children would not be able to assist in providing care for her.

Current Status

Imogene is using a walker to ambulate. She is physically able to prepare simple meals. The OT has been teaching her to bathe and dress herself c̄ adaptive equipment, so she can maintain her hip precautions for the next 3 weeks. Imogene had a great deal of difficulty learning the new tasks, and her safety awareness and judgment are poor. The nursing staff reports that in the evening, Imogene becomes very confused and it is difficult to calm her. The physician has indicated that Imogene has the initial symptoms of dementia.

Reimbursement Options

❏ home health care
❏ long-term care
❏ outpatient services

A. In your opinion, would Imogene benefit from further occupational therapy rehabilitative services?

B. What level of care would you recommend?

C. Provide an outline for a therapy plan that you would recommend for the next level of rehabilitative services you choose.

D. Would you recommend any type of community programs to the patient and her family?

EXERCISE 3:5 Alice

Alice is 20 y/o. She was involved in a diving accident that left her a paraplegic. Alice is very independent. She lives on her own and is working her way through college to be a pharmacist. She was employed as a waitress. Alice enjoys going to school and swimming.

Living Situation

Alice lived alone in an apartment prior to her injury. The injury occurred 2 months ago. Since then, her parents and sister moved her belongings to her parents' home. Alice's parents live in the family home, and her sister has an apt c̄ a roommate.

Phase of Recovery

Alice is in an inpatient rehab center that specializes in spinal cord injury recovery. Alice has received services c̄ OT, PT, and a psychologist.

Current Status

Alice is independent c̄ her self-care, transfers, and mobility in a lightweight w/c. Her strength and endurance are good. She has been reviewing her textbooks to catch up c̄ her studies and plans to return to school in 6 months.

Reimbursement Options

❏ home health services
❏ reentry programs
❏ outpatient services

A. In your opinion, would Alice benefit from further occupational therapy rehabilitative services?

B. What level of care would you recommend?

C. Provide an outline for a therapy plan that you would recommend for the next level of rehabilitative services you choose.

D. Would you recommend any type of community programs to the patient and her family?

Homer is 61 y/o. He had a heart attack 2 yrs ago, and he has DM. Three weeks ago, he had a BK amputation. Homer has always been very active. Prior to his heart attack, he worked as a salesman and did a lot of traveling. Since his heart attack, he decreased his travel schedule and volunteered as a radio operator for the fire department.

Phase of Recovery

Homer has been receiving OT and PT services in an amputee clinic for 2 weeks.

Living Situation

Homer lives c̄ his wife in a one-level condominium. They have a son who has a family and home. Homer assists his wife c̄ some of the household chores and takes care of the yard duties. Homer's wife is concerned about Homer's reaction to the amputation. He has indicated to her that he is useless s̄ his leg, even for volunteer work.

Current Status

Homer has received a LE prosthesis. He is ambulating independently c̄ a cane. He is indep c̄ dressing, bathing, and transfers c̄ his prosthesis. Homer is showing good weight-shifting ability, and he is able to monitor his stump skin condition. He went home on a weekend pass and reported he had no difficulties c̄ ambulating and self-care.

Reimbursement Options

❑ home health care
❑ reentry programs
❑ long-term care

A. In your opinion, would Homer benefit from further occupational therapy rehabilitative services?

B. What level of care would you recommend?

C. Provide an outline for a therapy plan you would recommend for the next level of rehabilitative services you choose.

D. Would you recommend any type of community programs to the patient and his family?

Stella is a 68 y/o F c̄ a Dx of COPD. She is being discharged to her home c̄ her husband. Stella is on oxygen 24 hours a day using a portable machine, and she uses a wheeled walker. She can walk about 30 ft and can perform activities for about 15 mins while sitting and then requires rest. She and her husband enjoy cooking and playing bridge.

The OTR has provided the following recommendations to prepare Stella for discharge:

❑ energy conservation guidelines
❑ bathroom, leisure, and adaptive kitchen equipment to conserve energy and ↑ functional activity
❑ list of activities pt can perform to maintain functional independence.

1. Provide a list of energy conservation guidelines that would be appropriate for Stella. Address the areas of self-care and leisure.

2. Provide a list of equipment recommendations you would like to offer Stella. Address areas of self-care in the bathroom and kitchen. Also, address leisure activities.

3. Provide Stella c̄ three activities that she can perform to maintain her sense of functional independence. (Remember her energy level.)

Mike is 48 y/o M who suffered a CHI 2° to an MVA. He will be d/c'd to his mother's home. His mother works during the day, so Mike will be left alone. Mike shows deficits c̄ his short-term memory, and he can sequence simple tasks such as putting together wood kits and birdhouses. His physical status is WFL.

The OTR has made the following recommendations for d/c:

❑ provide a list of safety considerations for the kitchen area 2° to ↓'d short-term memory
❑ provide a daily schedule/routine for Mike during the working day
❑ provide Mike and his mother c̄ leisure skills recommendations that involve the community (The mother is able to take him to activities in the evening.)

You are free to make assumptions regarding Mike's interests.

1. List the safety considerations you would need to consider for Mike in the kitchen area. Also list ways to resolve any problem areas you have identified.

2. List a daily routine for the hours of 8:30–5:00. Also provide a method to help Mike follow the routine.

3. List three options of community-based activities you can provide Mike and his mother.

DISCHARGE PROCESS AND HOME CARE

Erica is 57 y/o F c̄ a Dx of (L) CVA. She is being d/c'd to her home c̄ her husband. Her husband works during the day. Erica has no cognitive deficits. She has good sitting balance, but her standing balance and tolerance are fair. She can walk about 40 feet c̄ a LBQC. Her (R) hand is nonfunctional, and she is able to raise her arm about shoulder height c̄ effort, and can ✓ and / her elbow in gravity-eliminated positions. Erica is a homemaker. She has learned to dress and bathe herself in a rehabilitation hospital but requires equipment for going home.

The OTR has made the following recommendations for d/c:

❑ provide bathroom and kitchen equipment for safety and function
❑ recommend one-handed techniques for functional kitchen activities
❑ provide exercise program for (R) shoulder and elbow.

1. List the bathroom and kitchen equipment you would recommend. (Remember Erica does all the cooking.)

2. Describe three one-handed techniques Erica will need to be independent in the kitchen. (*Hint:* One can be how she can get items from one place to another; e.g., moving a pot from the stove to the sink.)

3. Provide a list and pictures of an exercise program for the following movements:

❑ shoulder flexion and extension against gravity
❑ shoulder adduction and abduction in gravity-eliminated positions
❑ elbow flexion and extension in gravity-eliminated positions
❑ elbow pronation and supination
❑ wrist flexion and extension in gravity-eliminated positions
❑ self-ROM for fingers and thumb.

(Practice explaining these exercises to a partner.)

Rita is 24 y/o F c̄ a Dx of (R) BKA 2° to diabetes. She is not a candidate for a prosthesis 2° to the fast progression of her disorder. Rita is also having difficulty c̄ her vision. She is safe for ambulation, but she is not able to drive or read items on signs. (*Example:* she is unable to read menus in fast-food restaurants.) Rita ambulates c̄ a walker; her endurance is good for short distances, but she is unable to manipulate stairs. Rita is a college student majoring in accounting. Most of her work is done on computers. She is independent c̄ bathing and dressing skills.

Rita is being d/c'd to her parents' home. Her plan is to return to college. Both her parents work, and their goal for Rita is to keep her as independent as possible. Rita is losing sensation in her hands. She will be able to continue using the computer, but she will not be able to learn Braille.

The OTR has provided the following recommendations for d/c:

❏ provide equipment recommendations for the bathroom area for safety and function
❏ provide recommendations for returning to school.

1. List equipment recommendations for the bathroom area.

2. List five problem areas Rita will likely encounter when she returns to school. Then provide recommendations on how they can be resolved. (The first area is provided for you.)

Problem: Transportation to and from school

Resolution:

Problem:

Resolution:

Problem:

Resolution:

Problem:

Resolution:

Problem:

Resolution:

References

Christiansen, C., & Baum, C. (1991). *Occupational therapy: Overcoming human performance deficits.* Thorofare, NJ: Slack.

DiMatteo, R. M. (1991). *The psychology of health, illness, and medical care.* Pacific Grove, CA: Brooks/Cole.

Appendix A

Common Medical Abbreviations

(A)	assisted
abd	abduction
ADL	activities of daily living
AFO	ankle-foot orthosis
AROM	active range of motion
ATNR	asymmetrical tonic neck reflex
(B)	both, bilateral
BF	black female
b.i.d.	two times daily
BKA	below-knee amputee
BM	black male
c̄	with
CHI	closed head injury
COTA	certified occupational therapist assistant
CT Scan	computed tomography scan
CVA	cerebrovascular accident
d/c	discharge
depend	dependent
DM	diabetes mellitus
doff	take off clothing
don	put on clothing
Dx	diagnosis
ECG	electrocardiogram (or: EKG)
EOM	edge-of-mat
ETOH	ethanol
eval	evaluation
exer	exercise
ext	extension
flex or ✓	flexion

fx	fracture
hemi	hemiplegia
(I)	independent
ICU	intensive care unit
IDDM	insulin-dependent diabetes mellitus
(L)	left
LE	lower extremity
LTG	long-term goals
max	maximal assistance
MI	myocardial infarction
min	minimal assistance
MMT	manual muscle test
MS	multiple sclerosis
MVA	motor vehicle accident
MVPT	motor free visual perception test
NG-tube	nasogastric tube
npo	nothing by mouth
OB helper	obstetrical aide
od	once daily
OOB	out of bed
OT	occupational therapy
Ox or O_2	oxygen
para	paraplegia
phys dys	physical dysfunction
p.r.n.	whenever necessary
PROM	passive range of motion
pt	patient
PT	physical therapy/physical therapist
(R)	right
RA	rheumatoid arthritis
rehab	Rehabilitation
s̄	without
SBA	standby assistance
SP	speech
s/p	status post
STG	short-term goals
STNR	symmetrical tonic neck reflex

sup	supination
THR	total hip replacement
TTWB	toe-touch weight bearing
tx	treatment/therapy
UE	upper extremities
UTI	urinary tract infection
WB	weight bearing
WBAT	weight bearing as tolerated
WBQC	wide-base quad cane
w/c	wheelchair
WF	white female
WFL	within functional limits
wk	week
WM	white male
y/n	yes/no
y/o	years old

Medical Symbols

(B)	both/bilateral
/	extension
F	fair
✓	flexion
G	good
N	normal
P	poor
2°	secondary
←	to the left
→	to the right
↔	to right and left or to and from
T	trace
c̄	with
s̄	without

Index